The
Parentalk
Guide to
Sleep

The
ParenTalk
Guide to
Sleep

The
ParenTalk
Guide to
Sleep

Kate Daymond

Series Editor: Steve Chalke

Illustrated by John Byrne

Hodder & Stoughton
LONDON SYDNEY AUCKLAND

British Library Cataloguing in Publication Data
A record for this book is available from the British Library

ISBN 0 340 78541 1

Typeset by Avon Dataset Ltd, Bidford-on-Avon, Warks

Printed and bound in Great Britain by
Clays Ltd, St Ives plc

Hodder and Stoughton
A Division of Hodder Headline Ltd
338 Euston Road
London NW1 3BH

Contents

Acknowledgements

There are many people behind a book like this and I'd like to thank the families who have generously shared their stories. I'd also like to express my gratitude to friends and colleagues, including the Buckley family, Dr Wendy Casey – Consultant Clinical Psychologist; Janice Fixter; Gerry McNeish; Dr John Tripp – Consultant Paediatrician and Senior Lecturer in Child Health at Exeter University; Dr Olwen Wilson – Clinical Psychologist – and her health visitor colleagues; and especially to Tim Mungeam for his encouragement and invaluable work.

'Haven't you finished your book yet, Mummy?' has been a frequent cry in our home, and my love and thanks go to Ella, Joe and Nick for their patience with my sleep obsession! Finally to my mum, Jenny Randall, whose care of Ella and Joe has meant writing this book has been possible; it is therefore dedicated to her, with my grateful thanks.

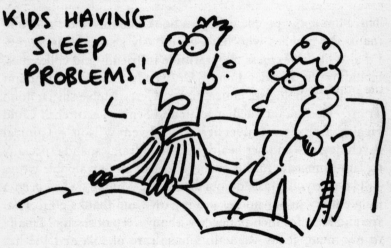

Introduction

Chances are, you won't have picked up this book if your child easily settles at bedtime and then sleeps like a lamb until 10 a.m. (and 11 a.m. at weekends). This is the kind of book you probably hoped that you would never have to read as your child grew up, but having faced night after night of interrupted sleep you're ready to try some ideas that have worked for other parents. On the other hand, you may be about to become a parent for the first time and, having been regaled with stories by your friends, have decided to try to get ahead of the competition!

Sleep problems aren't new. Generation after generation of mums and dads have patiently paced, rocked and soothed their infants well into the early hours – and beyond. Talk to any parent and they'll (more than likely) have an array of tricks and strategies they adopted to try and get their children to sleep. So there's every likelihood that the sleep problems that are driving you to distraction at the moment have also been faced by thousands of other mums and dads. But there's some good news. Not only are sleep difficulties experienced by lots of parents, but – given the right advice, reassurance and a large dose of courage – they are solved by lots of parents! And you can do it, too.

Psychologist Dr Spock (not the one with the pointy ears) told parents in the 1950s that 'you know more than you think you do'. And that's still the case today – what you do instinctively is often the best thing for your family. The trouble is, when you're struggling with a serious dose of sleep deprivation, it can be very hard to decide what the best thing is!

That's where the *Parentalk Guide to Sleep* can help. This book is a guide to the most common solutions to sleep problems – tried and tested by real parents. My aim has been to give you ideas that you can compare with your own situation, in the hope that it will help you to trust your instincts and build your confidence in tackling your family's sleep difficulties.

Sleep advice for the fashion-conscious

Like so many things in life, advice on sleep has gone through more fashions than *GQ* and *Cosmopolitan* put together. New suggestions have appeared with each generation. Reassuringly, like flared jeans, if you wait long enough each comes back into fashion eventually. Sleeping together with your baby, not sleeping with your baby, leaving him to cry, not leaving him to cry, using dummies, not using dummies, rocking to sleep ... the list is endless. It's hardly surprising that parents today feel uncertain! And that's part of the problem – children seem to thrive on parental confidence. Have you noticed that if you're the slightest bit unsure about how to get your child to sleep they'll sense it quicker than a hungry man at pub closing time sniffing out a kebab shop?

What's more, sleep advice varies according to the age of the child – so each chapter is written specifically with this in mind, highlighting the common difficulties experienced by children from birth to school, and providing ideas and tips on how to deal with them. For example, Chapters 3 and 4 explain how to avoid sleep problems in the first place by learning good sleep habits. Chapter 6 looks at the Seven Top Options for changing your child's sleep patterns, which means that it's one to make a beeline for, even if your child is older. Similarly, Chapter 9 tackles helping children sleep well in a variety of specific situations, regardless of their age (e.g. coping with the particular issues caused by childhood illnesses, multiple births and special needs).

 Top Tip: *What you do instinctively as a parent is often the best thing for your family.*

I'm not sure if I'm really ready . . .

One word of warning before we start. If you follow the advice in this book half-heartedly, it'll be a bit like attempting to start a diet when you know there's one of your favourite chocolate cakes in the fridge! You *must* be totally committed from the outset. For many new parents, their nights may be disturbed, but they simply are not ready for the challenge and commitment of working at changing their child's sleeping habits. If that sounds like you, put the search for an answer to sleep problems on the back burner for a while. When you're really fed up with getting no sleep and are desperate for your situation to change, pick up this book again and – take heart – you'll be a lot closer to having more sleep in your life!

Top Tip: *The more motivated you are to make things different, the more successful you will be.*

If you're ready to go for it now, though, sit in a comfy chair with a cup of tea and a chocolate Hobnob (that's my choice, but yours might be a beer and a bag of barbecue-flavour crisps) and come and see how other parents have faced up to the big issue of their child and sleep.

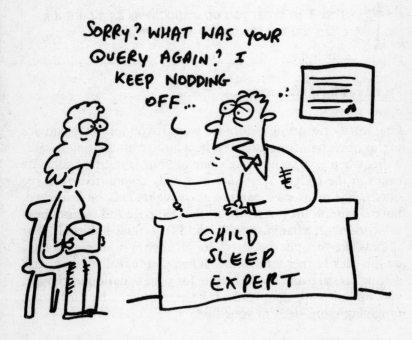

If You Don't Read Anything Else, Read This . . .

If you're just too tired to read this whole book then here's the edited highlights version:

★ Every parent has known what it is to be up in the night with their child – it's a standard part of parenting. I'm still up in the night sometimes with my two- and four-year-old even though I'm writing this book! So take heart. You are not the only one.

★ Some people fall asleep easily, others don't. Your child's personality inevitably plays a part in her sleep patterns, so don't automatically blame yourself if it's not going entirely according to plan straight away.

★ All children have a period of light sleep once every hour or so during the night, when they can be partially or completely awake.

★ You can't make your child sleep more than she needs – the important thing is that when she does sleep, she sleeps well.

★ If your child is a poor sleeper, even though she may appear to need very little sleep, it's likely she could sleep for much longer once she's learnt good sleep habits.

★ There are seven commonly used methods for solving sleep problems, explained fully in Chapter 6, that are suitable for children from three months old to school age.

★ If you have a partner, it's important you both agree on any new plans for bedtime and night-time. All of us like to know what's expected of us in certain situations, and sending 'mixed messages' to your child will only result in confusion, not success.

★ Decide on some *realistic* first steps you can take in your particular circumstances that will ensure your family's nights are how you'd like them to be. Once you're motivated and ready, take the decision to start. It may take some time to reach your final objective (anything from three nights to three months), but it *will* be worth it.

★ How your child learns to fall asleep at bedtime is how she'll want to fall asleep when she wakes in the night. If your baby has fallen asleep in your arms, for example, she will want to be held again to fall back to sleep during the night. If she has learnt to fall asleep without you at bedtime she is more likely to fall back to sleep on her own in the night.

★ Bed-sharing is a common short-term solution to a tiny screaming newborn baby at 3 a.m., because she is more likely to settle when close to you. However, it's not safe to sleep with your baby if:

• you or your partner smoke,

- you have been drinking,
- you have been taking drugs that make you drowsy, or
- you are excessively tired (see Chapter 4 for lots more detail).

While the link between cot death and having your baby in bed with you is still unclear, recommendations from the Department of Health err on the side of caution and suggest that while your baby is young, she sleeps in her own cot as much as possible, in your room.

★ Every family is different. One will be content sharing beds for several years, another will want their child in a separate room as soon as possible. What is important is to decide early on where you really want your child to sleep and to work hard towards achieving that goal.

★ Don't be 'brave' – call on friends and family as much as you can to help you through the rough patches. If you're worried about your child, seek the advice of your health visitor or doctor.

★ Take it easy on yourself – you're probably doing much better than you think. Regardless of what anyone tells you, even seasoned parents have their L-plates firmly attached – the trick is to make sure that we learn from our mistakes.

★ Both you and your child are individuals, so no standard advice will ever fit your unique situation perfectly. Therefore, take the advice in this book that feels instinctively right for you and fits your needs, and forget the rest.

★ With perseverance and dedication, your situation will change for the better. Millions of parents have already cracked it, and you can too!

 Top Tip: *If you don't have time to read the whole book, read this chapter again.*

Birth to Three Months

Your baby has arrived. The congratulations cards with pictures of smiling contented babies are taking up every surface, and you feel . . . totally exhausted, like nothing on earth. Why didn't someone tell you how tired you'd be? 'All-nighters' used to mean music, dancing till dawn and a long lie-in, not smelly nappies, incessant crying and work in the morning.

Like the calm before the storm, the day of his actual birth will probably see your new baby spending most of it asleep. However, even at this earliest of stages, new mums and dads can find themselves getting anxious. Try not to. Your baby needs the rest, and you do, too! Whether you are mum or dad, even the most straightforward labour will have left you feeling exhausted, so give your new family the time it needs to recover, readjust and sleep while you can.

Is there a money-back guarantee?

From then on, for most people, getting through the early weeks is a case of survival and doing what comes naturally. It's been said that raising children is part joy, part guerrilla warfare, and the early days may see you feeling frazzled and with little confidence. If your baby is irritable and unsettled at this stage, it's unlikely that it's anything that you're doing that is making him restless, but far more likely to do with who he is and what he's been through. Try not to blame yourself unnecessarily – just do what you can to provide reassurance in the form of cuddles or whatever he seems to enjoy most.

Top Tip: *Make the most of your chances to catch up on lost sleep – sleep when your baby does. It might seem anti-social, but in the long term it's well worth it!*

Getting night and day the right way round

Babies tend to be born with a nocturnal clock, and as a result are often very perky in the middle of the night. You can help your baby gradually change his orientation by adopting the tried and tested 'I'm positively boring to be with at night but a top entertainer in the day' approach. Of course, to a certain extent nature already does this for you – if you're already tired, any possibility of raising a smile during the night will have probably been lost a week or so ago!

Top Tip: *You can help your baby get night and day the right way round by being positively boring to be with at night!*

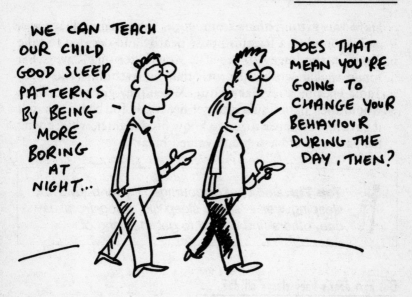

It's a relief to know that before the age of three months your baby can't really learn any bad habits. It means you can feel free to experiment with different ways of getting him off to sleep. You could join the 3 a.m. night-time drivers' club, rock him to sleep, have a bath together or hold him close in bed while he feeds. Some babies like being swaddled in a sheet, others hate it. Some like being put down in their cots and left to get to sleep, while others seem to fight any feelings of tiredness with every ounce of energy they can muster.

Dave was overwhelmed with joy when his first child, Tania, was born, but he quickly discovered that he couldn't stand her crying. Most days Tania would become miserable just as

11

Dave was getting home from work. One evening Dave was going round to a friend's house nearby and decided to take Tania in the buggy to see if it would stop her crying. He found that it worked so well that his evening walks with Tania became a regular fixture. When they got home, Dave would then bath Tania and get her ready for bed. Dave felt it gave him a chance to get to know his daughter, while giving his partner Debbie a much-valued break.

 Top Tip: Don't get discouraged if your baby's not sleeping well – some sleep like a log from day one, others find it hard to get the hang of.

But next door's baby sleeps all day . . .

Most newborns drift in and out of sleep during the day and night, feeding little and often. But as they become more established, somewhere around the age of six weeks, they tend to wake up more and need to feed roughly every two to four hours. During this period they can sleep in between feeds for anything up to several hours or for as little as twenty minutes. On the whole, though, babies less than three months old generally sleep for about sixteen or seventeen hours out of every twenty-four.

Do your best to avoid comparing your own baby's sleeping pattern with the experiences of other parents – you'll either be disheartened or end up feeling so smug that you lose all your friends who are still struggling. The truth is that your baby is unique. Every baby is different – each one needs different amounts of sleep. If you ask around you'll discover that there is a wide range of 'normal', and your baby's sleeping habits probably fit well within it.

Top Tip: *Every baby is different, so get to know your own baby's sleeping habits rather than just looking at how much other babies sleep.*

He's awake – he must be hungry!

Feeding and sleeping tend to go hand in hand at this stage, so you'll probably find yourself thinking that your baby must be hungry if he wakes. As we will see later, however, babies wake up for all sorts of reasons – and most like to suck even when they are full up. But, in truth, babies are more likely to sleep well if they are left to build up an appetite in readiness for a longer, more satisfying feed. If they get into the habit of snacking on small amounts every hour, they are unlikely to sleep for long in between. Unless your midwife or health visitor recommends otherwise, over the next few weeks try not to feed your baby any more than two-hourly. For example, if you start feeding him at 7 a.m., try not to offer another feed until 9 a.m.

Top Tip: *Babies tend to sleep for longer if they have a good feed every few hours, rather than little 'snack' feeds every twenty minutes.*

Eyes wide open

As the weeks go by, your baby will spend more time awake in between feeds and will gradually become more interested in the world around him. He may wake earlier but not be ready for a feed. Instead, he may want some stimulation – looking at your face, watching tree branches moving in the wind or looking at mobiles against the light.

If you haven't caught up on your sleep by the time your baby is four to six weeks old, the reality is that you'll have less opportunity as time goes by. So, however hard you may find it and however tempting it may be to get on with the household chores, the golden rule is to try and rest as much as possible in these early days. Try to sleep (or at least rest) when your baby sleeps – even a snatched ten minutes will make a difference.

 Top Tip: *In the early days, try to forget the housework for a while and snatch some sleep while your baby sleeps.*

Feeding and sleeping – the dynamic duo

By six weeks, most babies are feeding three or four times a night. Typically, your baby might want to spend a long time feeding in the evening and, just when you think he's had enough, he'll have another bottle or breast feed at 8 or 9 p.m. He might then sleep until midnight or 1 a.m., waking for another feed, and then again at 4 or 5 a.m., and again at 7 or 8 a.m.

Of course, as you'll probably have guessed by now, in the same way as with so much of parenthood, none of this is written in stone. Your baby might be feeding much less than this during the night, which means you can relax and read all this with a satisfied expression all over your face! On the other hand, many babies of this age will still be waking every couple of hours or so throughout the night. And the truth is, both are entirely normal!

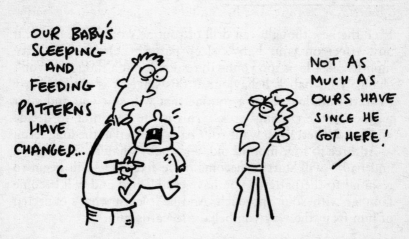

OUR BABY'S SLEEPING AND FEEDING PATTERNS HAVE CHANGED...

NOT AS MUCH AS OURS HAVE SINCE HE GOT HERE!

The golden rule in these early weeks is not to get too hung up if even your best-laid plans for his feeding and sleeping regime don't work out.

As babies grow, their feeding and sleeping patterns change – they can go for longer without the need for food. As the night feeds drop, you will slowly discover again how delicious it is to be able to sleep for more than three hours at a time.

Top Tip: *Don't try and plan his feeding and sleeping too much in the early weeks – just as your baby gets settled into one routine, he may well change his habits.*

When is it good to start routines?

Even the best thought-out drill or routine won't have much, if any, effect on your baby's sleep pattern before he is three months old – he is too young to respond. But although it won't change your baby's behaviour at this stage, it is not too early to start thinking about a routine that will suit you and your partner in the coming weeks. This is the best time to decide how (and where) you want your baby to sleep in the long term.

At three to four months old, your baby's habits – both good and bad – will start to become more fixed. He will begin to respond to the patterns you have established and will become familiar with your approach. And he'll learn what's expected of him from the way you behave towards him.

Some lucky parents produce babies who fall into a natural sleep pattern on their own. Babies of eight weeks who sleep for six to eight hours in the night (at convenient times) are the envy of every other parent. But for those mums and dads who are less fortunate and whose three-month-olds don't just slip into these marvellous habits (and there are plenty of us!), it's important to begin to create some boundaries and structure which will help them to sleep well in the long run. Try to decide now which habits you want to encourage and which habits you want to avoid, so that you can be as ready as possible.

> **Top Tip:** At three to four months old, your baby's habits will start to become fixed – good and bad. Now's the time to consider which ones you want to encourage.

The terrible two: coping with crying and colic

Crying and colic are the most likely causes of persistent sleep disturbance – for both you and your baby – in the first three months.

Crying

Living with a crying baby is debilitating, emotionally draining and isolating. During the first three months, some babies can seem to cry all day long; they fuss and whine and are generally miserable. Others just target peak times to fill their lungs, scream and holler. Though not very pleasant at the best of times, if you're already tired a howling baby can feel like more than you can cope with.

If nothing you do seems to console him, your frustration can easily spill over, which of course will make him even more anxious because you're not smiling sweetly at him any more. The vicious circle is then complete and you can go round and round it together, dragging each other down for weeks. Aaaaaghaghaaagh!

Checkpoint Charlie

Of course, a crying baby is also unlikely to sleep well, and as a result will test the patience of any parent to the absolute limit. As his mum or dad, it's easy to feel there must be something that you're doing wrong which has caused all this to happen, and that it's therefore all your fault. However, this is simply not true – so don't be too hard on yourself.

Though your baby's sleep problems are very unlikely to be down to anything you've done, there might be some positive things that you can do to help him settle. Ask yourself whether he is:

- excessively wet or has a dirty nappy which needs changing;
- over-tired or over-stimulated – have you had lots of visitors?
- too hot or too cold;
- generally unwell – does he have any other symptoms?
- hungry or thirsty (if he is genuinely thirsty he'll drink cooled-down boiled water);

- windy, uncomfortable or suffering from 'gripey' tummy pains (if so, stroke his tummy gently in a clockwise circle, with some baby oil on your hands);
- bored and wanting to be entertained;
- wanting to be held – does he quieten as soon as you pick him up?
- wanting to be left alone – sometimes too much interference can make the situation worse, not better;
- wanting to suck, even though he isn't hungry. It's worth trying a dummy – it could be really useful in the early weeks (see page 57 for more on the pros and cons of dummies).

If none of these possibilities seems to provide you with an answer, don't hesitate to talk to your health visitor or doctor. Be reassured, though, that as your baby grows you'll find it easier to work out what's going on and what works for him.

If all else fails and your baby is still very restless and finding it hard to fall asleep after feeds at night-time, he is much more likely to be comforted if he is close to you and kept as undisturbed as possible. But remember, it's not safe to let your baby sleep with you if either you or your partner are smokers (even if you do not smoke in bed), if either partner has been drinking or taking drugs that make you drowsy, or if you are excessively tired. (For more information, see the advice on sleeping safely with your baby on page 36.)

 Top Tip: *The more you get to know your baby, the better you'll get at working out the reasons for him crying.*

Rock around the clock

In the 1800s, rocking your crying baby became very trendy – so much so that the well-to-do employed professional 'rockers' to do it for them. One parenting manual published in 1755 had four pages dedicated to the art of rocking a cradle! We now know, from recent research, just how good all that rocking was for those babies. But we also now know that distressed babies calm down even more quickly if they are rocked lying flat in your arms, continuously at a reasonable speed – in fact it has even been scientifically discovered that the speed of a traditional rocking chair is perfect!

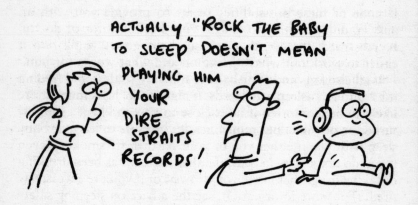

ACTUALLY "ROCK THE BABY TO SLEEP" DOESN'T MEAN PLAYING HIM YOUR DIRE STRAITS RECORDS!

Don't expect your baby to be completely quiet all the time. Even the most contented babies cry some of the time. But few new parents appreciate that this crying can often be a healthy sign.

Will someone please keep the noise down!
Babies can be very sensitive to noise. Some like absolute peace and quiet, while others are frightened if it's too quiet – they like to hear people talking, loos flushing and the sound of the radio in the background. Remember, your baby has been getting used to hearing your voice while in the womb and so will find the sounds in your home comforting. Generally, babies prefer background noises rather than sudden loud ones. For example, they won't wake up when the washing machine is on but they might if you bang the front door.

And, of course, babies themselves can often be quite noisy at night. In fact, it can be incredibly frustrating when your child sleeps well himself but the noise he makes keeps you awake. The Foundation of the Study of Infant Death (FSID) recommends that babies should sleep in the same room with you for the first six months, even though some parents find this advice hard to follow. A noisy baby can be so difficult to sleep with – it's a bit like having a hedgehog in a paper bag rustling around the room! So take a look at all the recommendations (coming up in the next chapter) and try to follow as many as you can.

Colic

Colic is often the cause of disturbed sleep and screaming in babies under four months old, and most normally occurs in the evening. Though there are breast-fed and bottle-fed babies all over the world suffering from colic, unfortunately no one really knows either the cause or the treatment. Talk to your health visitor if your baby is suffering and get their advice.

21

Though colic won't damage your baby, it is likely to frazzle your nerves and confidence. A baby with colic typically draws his knees up to his tummy, clenches his fists and screams without any consolation for a fixed time every night. He may cry for several hours, usually at least three or four nights a week, lasting several weeks. Most parents' natural reaction is to pick the baby up and rock him continuously, changing position frequently as the crying persists. However, the most recent research indicates that babies with colic tend to settle more quickly when they are handled and rocked less. So if you haven't tried it yet, let your baby have a rest in his cot for a while rather than spending long periods rocking, patting and pacing – the less stimulation the better.

Sometimes colic can be linked to a baby's difficulty in digesting cow's milk. To test this, your GP or health visitor might suggest a diet free of cow's milk for a maximum of two weeks. It's important, however, that you only do this with their support so they can make sure your baby doesn't miss out on any vital nutrients.

Colic usually stops around the age of four months, for no apparent reason and as quickly as it came (although some experts believe that this may be because the gut has become more mature). Here are some tips that have helped soothe other parents and babies through this hard time and that may also help you:

- Watch what your baby responds to best – he might prefer less stimulation rather than more.
- Play monotonous sounds – like a hairdryer or washing machine (a home-made tape-recording of the vacuum

cleaner worked for one dad, the sound of running water for another). This can help your baby become less alert to his surroundings, and less irritable as a result.

- Play music – continuous playing of Steps, Duke Ellington and opera have all been known to help.
- Gentle, rhythmical movements seem to help some babies – does he enjoy being in a sling, or pushed in the pram?
- Give him skin-to-skin contact when you do pick him up – babies love this sensation, and the sound of your heartbeat will have a reassuring, calming effect.
- Ask your pharmacist about the products that you can buy over the counter – gripe water, colic drops, etc. Most people give them a try because they are so desperate to relieve the crying, and they do work for some.
- Ask your health visitor for advice about testing for cow's milk intolerance.

One final thought about colic – the parents I've known who've got through the first few months looking after a baby with colic have certainly honed up their patience skills, which all comes in handy later on!

 Top Tip: _Colic won't damage your baby, but it is likely to frazzle your nerves and confidence. Remember, it will stop before too long._

'Something's not right'

At the end of the day, if you have tried everything you can think of and have still been unable to settle your crying baby, don't hesitate to seek advice from your health visitor or GP. Parents often have a sixth sense when something is not right – they know it deep down. Trust your instinct. Most doctors and nurses have little blue lights at the back of their heads that start flashing when parents present their baby to them saying, 'I don't know what it is, but something's not right.'

> **Top Tip:** If you're convinced that something's not right – even if you don't know what it is – don't hesitate to contact your GP or health visitor. Trust your instinct.

What can I do when my baby won't stop crying?

★ Use a soft voice and calming words, looking straight into his eyes. As difficult as it may be, try to look calm!
★ Try stroking and gentle massage when he starts becoming miserable (and before he's hollering for England).
★ Remind yourself that it's unlikely to be anything you're doing wrong – your baby just needs as much reassurance as you can give.

★ If you are on your own and you've run out of patience and empathy, put the baby in a safe place (like his cot) and spend a few minutes away from his cries.

★ Do whatever is safe and minimises his distress – whether it's cuddling in bed together (see health advice on page 36), carrying him in a sling, driving round the block at 3 a.m., using a dummy, watching television together, listening to music, rocking him, or taking him outside and pointing out what you can see.

★ Recent research shows that too much intervention can make the situation worse rather than better. So think about whether there is anything that you could stop doing!

The first three months of a baby's life can be just about the hardest for the new mum or dad, especially if he finds it hard to settle. Try not to let it get to you, however – though you may not believe it at the time, things *will* get better.

 Top Tip: *Though you may not believe it at the time, things will get better! So go easy on yourself – you may not realise how well you're coping.*

Left holding the baby

When you travel on a plane, a member of the cabin crew always carefully explains what to do in case of a 'loss in cabin pressure'. 'An oxygen mask will drop down automatically from a compartment above your head: place it over your head, secure the straps, and breathe normally.' But there's a little extra instruction for parents: fasten your own mask before trying to fasten your child's mask. The reason they have to be so emphatic about this point is because, as we all know, most parents would naturally help out their child before taking care of themselves. But in fact, trying to fit an oxygen mask over the head of a frightened, perhaps even panic-stricken, child is difficult and often time-consuming. If a parent is struggling for breath at the same time as trying to fit their child's mask, the result is likely to be disastrous for both of them.

This 'oxygen mask principle' also extends to the rest of the parent's life. So as you look at the 24-hour clock that makes up your day, don't forget to put in time for yourself and time with your partner if you have one. The mistake some parents make is to spend virtually every waking moment either working or caring for their child, without creating or protecting a little 'oasis' of time for themselves. As a result, they're almost permanently exhausted and never really feel on top of things. The irony is, this isn't an efficient way of coping. In fact, it isn't really a way of coping at all.

So it's important you catch up on lost sleep during your baby's sleep times, particularly if you are bringing up the baby on your own. If you can't really get to sleep in the day – and

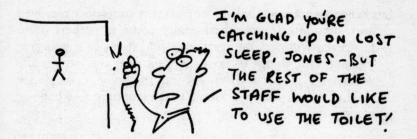

I'M GLAD YOU'RE CATCHING UP ON LOST SLEEP, JONES – BUT THE REST OF THE STAFF WOULD LIKE TO USE THE TOILET!

many parents find it hard to switch off – even a couple of ten-minute catnaps can make a huge difference. You may even begin to see the return of a friend you thought was lost for ever – your sense of humour!

Here are some ways to sneak some rest into your day:

- *Not dressing to impress*
  Just occasionally in the first six weeks, try wearing pyjamas all day. Although some people's personalities mean that they always feel better once they're dressed, for me it had a brilliant effect. For instance, visitors are more likely to make their own cups of tea, and might even wash up their own mug! If you're not only dressed but also looking pristine and smelling of expensive perfume, then they may well think you're coping successfully enough to look after *them* as well as a new baby. (And they won't even dare to ask if they can do anything to help if you're looking that organised!)

- *You need friends . . .*
  Take up offers of help whenever you can. This is where

grandads, grannies, half-brothers, great aunts once removed and anyone else you trust really come into their own. However, willing volunteers may find it easier if you give them specific things to do – i.e. look after the baby while you have a proper shower, vacuum the home, cook a nice meal, or take a sack of washing to the laundrette – whatever is most important to you.

- ### *This season, the dusty look is 'in'*
  Try to lower your expectations of how clean your home is when visitors arrive. You could write 'I know it's dusty' in the dust on the mantelpiece or show them where you keep the Hoover if they look disapproving! If, however, you really can't bear an untidy home and all it does is add to your stress, make a list of the things which you really want to get done and just tick off one or two a day.

- ### *For goodness sake, SIT DOWN!*
  If you simply can't sleep when your baby does, at least make yourself sit down, listen to your favourite music, read a magazine and chill. Drifting off on the sofa for ten minutes is restorative, and a twenty-minute 'power nap' is great: Japanese businessmen swear by them, and if *they* need them, then do you really need me to convince you that you need one too?

- ### *Get an early night*
  Another big way of recouping some long stretches of sleep in these early months is to go to bed when your baby has had his last feed in the evening. I'm a 'can't do with less

than nine hours a night' sort of sleeper, so friends soon gave up calling us after 9 p.m. when our son was born because they knew we'd be in bed. And knowing that I could have four hours' uninterrupted sleep was more precious to me than watching yet another repeat of *Fawlty Towers* or *Friends*.

For some, though, the thought of an early-to-bed regime is totally abhorrent. So if you can't face dramatically losing your social life even for a short period, why not try having three or four early nights a week – you'll find it makes a big difference, and on the other evenings you can still party all you like! But remember, the sleep you lose each night will have a cumulative effect; grabbing sleep when you can will keep your body from becoming chronically sleep-deprived and so protect you from what can be the severe effects of that situation.

- *You are what you eat*
  Eat well and eat regularly, as this will help with fatigue. If you are breast-feeding, it will also ensure that your milk is satisfying in terms of nutrients and quantity for the baby, which may in turn mean he'll sleep better. Even if you're not, though, if you're at home on your own with the baby you'll find there is a big temptation to skip your meals. So watch out. You're never going to be able to look after him properly if you're having breakfast at 3 p.m.!

- *Snack attack*
  Ask friends, relatives or the supermarket online direct delivery man to bring you a big plate of your favourite

sandwiches (even if it is honey and Marmite with pickled onions). Stick them in the fridge and nibble them when you get two minutes to yourself. Other quick nutritious food ideas are cereal, packets of dried fruit (apricots, pears, raisins), toast with cheese, cold meats, pâté and bananas. I know you'll already be tucking into the Mars bars and crisps, so there's no point in mentioning those!

Top Tip: *If you can't sleep when your baby does, at least make yourself sit down, listen to your favourite music, have a drink, read a magazine and chill.*

The first three months – SURVIVAL!

Some would say that, however beautifully behaved your baby, the first few weeks of parenthood are among the toughest you'll experience. But parents of a restless baby can feel particularly deflated, hopeless, incoherent and disorientated. If you do, don't feel guilty – it's normal and it's probably a passing phase.

As long as it's safe, find anything that helps you and your baby to sleep as much as possible, and stick with it. It's too early for your baby to really learn any bad sleeping habits yet, but as you get nearer the end of the third month, remember to start thinking about where you want everyone to sleep. Getting your baby's feeding established goes hand in hand with sleeping well, so if you find everything is going pear-shaped with feeding get some advice from your baby clinic and your health visitor. Do it sooner rather than later – visiting your baby clinic will also give you the chance to meet other parents in similar situations to yours.

Whether you're Mum or Dad, you need time to get to know your baby and he needs to get to know you. You've never met before, so give it a bit of time! Go easy on yourself and stock up with lots of good videos and frozen pizzas.

 Top Tip: *In the early days, take time to get to know your baby and to recover yourself. Don't worry too much about the housework or establishing the perfect sleep pattern quite yet!*

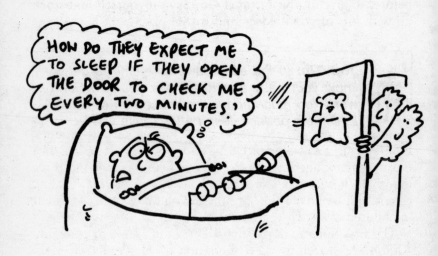

Sudden Infant Death Syndrome - Reducing the Risk

One of the biggest fears that every parent faces is that their baby will stop breathing in the night. If you're already a parent, how many times have you quickly 'just checked' to see that your baby is OK? Babies who die completely unexpectedly, for no apparent reason, are described as having suffered Sudden Infant Death Syndrome (SIDS), also known as cot death. The most common age for this to occur is between two and three months – it becomes less common as babies get older, being rare in children over nine months old and almost non-existent in children over two years of age.

The first thing to say about SIDS is that it is not common. Although research by the Foundation for the Study of Infant Deaths has found that an average of eight babies per week in the UK die as a result of SIDS, this is still a very small percentage of the total number of births. Yet just one death would still be too many, and so a great deal of energy has been put into researching the causes of SIDS.

Top Tip: *Cot death is not common, but it is still important to do everything you can to minimise the risk.*

It might not stop you worrying, but there are five important steps you can take to provide as much protection as possible for your baby.

1 *Back to sleep and feet to foot*
   Unless your midwife or doctor gives you a specific reason not to, always *put your baby to sleep lying on her back.* Her feet should also be touching the bottom of the cot or Moses basket so that she can't wriggle further down the bed and end up with the blankets covering her head. In the same way, because they can easily slip over her head, duvets and quilts aren't regarded as safe for babies under a year, and pillows aren't safe until she's two years old. Additionally, always use cotton blankets that you can tuck in and never put a hat on your baby to sleep in even if she is cold.

2 *Smoke-free zone*
   There is a proven link between cot death and smoking. Research suggests that the number of deaths from SIDS would be reduced by almost two-thirds if parents didn't smoke, and so the best advice is to quit. Of course, as the saying goes, 'giving up smoking is easy – I've done it thousands of times'! If you can't give it up, be encouraged that there are still important things you can do to lower the risk to your baby:

- Always smoke well away from your baby (never in the same room) and ensure any visitors do the same.
- Cut down the number of cigarettes you smoke. Ask yourself as you pull a cigarette out of the packet, 'Do I really need to smoke this now or could I wait a while?'
- Make sure you get some good support if you're trying to cut down or stop smoking. See the Quitline telephone number at the back of this book.

If you do smoke, a cigarette can be the only thing that keeps you going after a bad night of disrupted sleep. So work out where you can have the smoke you need, while also making sure that your baby's health is not harmed by the smoke you exhale.

 Top Tip: *Get a balance between your baby's needs and your own – you're important too!*

3 *Not too hot*

Don't let your baby get too hot. After coping with sub-tropical temperatures in hospital it's natural to feel your home should be just as hot, and certainly warm enough for you to walk around in your underwear! However, as your baby gets older she'll also become less vulnerable. It is far healthier to let her adjust to the normal temperatures of your home. Try and get a feel of how hot or cold she becomes during the night. Never judge the warmth of your baby by her hands or feet, as they tend always to be cool.

Feel her head or tummy instead, as this will give you a much truer idea of her temperature. Young babies are not able to adjust their body temperature well, so will quickly get hot if wrapped up too much (or cold if not wrapped up enough).

Our natural instinct is to prevent babies from getting too cold. In fact, most babies are more at risk from becoming too hot – especially if Great Aunt Ethel's knitted an extra snugly double-ply blanket that she's expecting to see being used when popping by unannounced. So don't leave heating on overnight in your baby's room, unless it's really wintry in there. The general rule is (day or night) that babies need the same as you're wearing with one more layer, and the room where they sleep should be between 16 and 20° Centigrade.

4 *Prompt medical advice*
If your baby is unwell, especially with a raised temperature or breathing difficulties, and/or is less responsive than normal, do go and see a doctor promptly. You know your child better than anyone else, and if your intuition is telling you something isn't right, listen and act on it.

5 *Bed-sharing for comfort, not sleep*
Some studies show that bed-sharing is beneficial to a baby's health, others link it with SIDS. Current thinking is that the research neither proves nor disproves a link between bed-sharing and the health of the baby, so the latest Department of Health advice errs on the side of caution. They recognise that many parents do share beds with their baby,

especially to feed or to give her comfort, but they recommend that you *put her back into her own cot or Moses basket to sleep*.

One conclusion of the research which is clear, however, is that you should never share your bed with your baby if you:

- have drunk alcohol;
- smoke (even if you don't actually smoke in bed);
- are taking any medicines or drugs which make you drowsy;
- are feeling excessively tired.

If you choose to have your baby in bed with you (and many parents do), be aware of the following advice:

- Make sure your partner knows the baby is in the bed.
- Make sure your baby is away from your pillows, the duvet or bedclothes, and not likely to roll off the bed!
- Remember that, when sleeping in the family bed, your baby has a warm parent's body (or two) nearby. It's therefore important not to overdress her.

Basic common sense really, but this is the most up-to-date advice currently available. Of course, it may change as more is discovered about the causes of SIDS, so listen out for any new developments. If you're concerned or unsure about anything, seek further advice from your health visitor.

Top Tip: Follow the five steps to reducing the chances of cot death:

- Back to sleep and feet to foot
- Smoke-free zone
- Not too hot
- Prompt medical advice
- Bed-sharing for comfort, not sleep.

Waterbeds, sofas and mattresses

If you have a waterbed (lucky you), don't be tempted to let your baby sleep on it at any time. Young babies and children can easily get stuck face down on the mattress and will be unable to reposition themselves.

Recent research has also shown that it's not safe to fall asleep with your baby in your arms on the sofa. However tempting it is to drift off together in front of a late-night film, make sure you put her down first before you doze off. Never leave it to chance.

In the early 1990s there was a scare linking SIDS with the chemicals in PVC cot-mattress covers. However, more recent research shows that there is now no evidence to indicate any link. Current recommendations are that you use a mattress with a firm flat surface: one that is clean, dry and well aired. Even if a cot mattress has ventilation holes at the head, always place your baby at the foot of the bed (the feet-to-foot position) to avoid overheating.

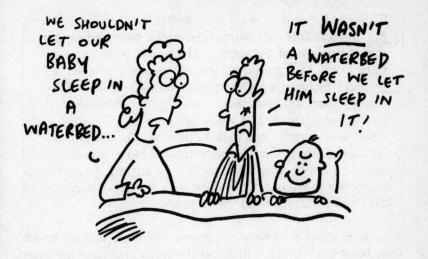

Baby monitors, apnoea alarms and things that go 'beep' in the night

There are a growing number of baby gadgets you can buy these days, including an alarming (excuse the pun) array of monitors that won't disappoint even the keenest gismo addict.

A baby monitor is really useful if you have put your baby in another room and can't hear her cry from other parts of your home. Some monitors have volume switches, so you don't have to listen to the crying – they merely flash lights at you when your baby makes a noise. But though monitors in themselves are obviously helpful, it still all comes down to the way they are used . . .

Sarah, fed up with always hearing her baby cry in the night, put the monitor on Tony's side of the bed, and he agreed that the next time the baby cried it would be his turn to sort things out. Half an hour later the monitor relayed a loud shriek, which woke Sarah up. She waited a while and looked over to Tony, who was still fast asleep. She decided not to go to the baby herself and woke Tony up to tell him that the baby was crying and that he had to do something. He groaned, lifted his hand slowly up over to the monitor – and switched it off. That was his way of sorting it. And what happened to the baby? She cried for a few more minutes and then went back to sleep on her own.

The latest trend is to have an apnoea alarm – a mat on which your baby lies while she sleeps. If she stops breathing for more than a specific length of time an alarm goes off. In a healthy child with no family history of SIDS, it could be argued that the anxiety involved in listening for it to go off can outweigh the benefits. Studies conducted by the Foundation for the Study of Infant Deaths (see their details at the back of the book for more information) have found no evidence that alarms help to prevent cot death. You may choose to use an apnoea alarm if it makes you worry less, but never let it lull you into a false sense of security by making you less vigilant.

So, to recap – we know these five steps do reduce the risk of cot death, so follow as many of them as you can:

- Put your baby to sleep on her back, in the feet-to-foot position.
- Quit smoking – mothers and fathers too!

- Don't let your baby get too hot – always keep her head uncovered.
- If your baby is unwell ask for a doctor's advice promptly.
- Bed-share for feeding and comfort, but let your baby sleep in her own cot.

Three to Six Months

You've now reached the stage where your baby's personality will be really beginning to shine through. He will start taking solid food when he's between four and six months old, which in itself may help him settle and sleep better at night. Some three- or four-month-old babies are still feeding two to three times in the night, while others need just one feed and some don't need any.

Babies between three and six months tend to sleep for up to sixteen hours out of twenty-four, with a couple of daytime sleeps (usually one in the morning and one in the afternoon).

Five-and-a-half-month-old Gaby has recently dropped her 4 a.m. feed, much to the delight of both her parents. This is an example of her typical feeding and sleeping pattern for one day:

6.40 a.m.	Wakes up
8.00 a.m.	Breakfast – 5oz bottle-feed and a few spoons of cereal
10.00 – 11.00 a.m.	Morning sleep – sleeps in her cot, crying for five to ten minutes when initially put down
11.00 a.m.	3–5oz bottle-feed

1.00 p.m.	Lunch – mashed potato and carrot, 3oz bottle-feed
2.00 – 4.00 p.m.	Afternoon sleep
4.00 p.m.	5oz bottle-feed
6.30 p.m.	Supper – fruit puree with baby rice
7.30 p.m.	Bedtime drink – 4oz bottle-feed before going to sleep
11.30 p.m.	Wakes for 5oz bottle-feed, settles back to sleep on her own

You mean it's normal for him to wake up in the night?

All of us, children and adults alike, 'wake' several times during the night. As we rest, we go through different stages of what's known as the sleep cycle, a cycle which is repeated over and over again throughout the night. The light sleep stage occurs when we relax and first fall asleep. Then we move into the restorative part of sleep where we dream – known in the trade as REM (not the pop group). This stands for Rapid Eye Movement because our eyes move a lot while we dream. The very deep sleep stage comes next – this is when even a herd of elephants marching through your home – and doing the hoovering as they went – wouldn't wake you up. We dream again before moving back into light sleep, and so the cycle begins again.

If you're woken up while you are dreaming it leaves you disorientated, woozy and feeling rotten. If, on the other hand, you wake during your light period of sleep, in theory at least you feel more alert. A baby waking during the light sleep stage will wake up happier, too!

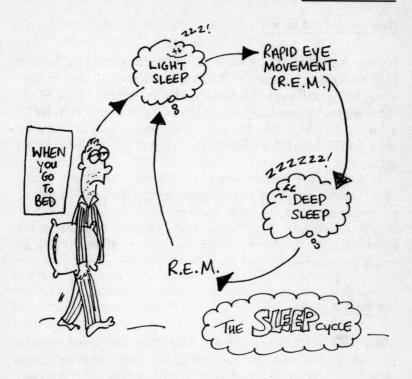

Babies and children have many more light sleep periods than adults. In babies, each cycle lasts around sixty minutes, and so they will experience periods of light sleep roughly every hour each night. These are the times when your baby may wake up and cry – when he realises he isn't still in your arms on the sofa watching *Match of the Day*.

Make your bed and lie in it

Now is the time to think seriously about the word you'll either love or hate – 'routines'! This is a good time to decide how your family will sleep: all in bed together, separate beds in the same room, in separate rooms? If you have a choice, don't be afraid to do what's best for you – if you're getting enough sleep then you'll be able to look after your baby without being grumpy!

If you have a partner, do you both want the same thing? Have you had a chance to talk about it with them? Try to agree on a way forward that suits you both. If one of you feels that they're losing out, it will only makes things much harder for everyone and put added pressure on your relationship. Try, as much as possible, to look for a 'win–win' situation.

The choice is yours

There are lots of things you can do to help your child learn to fall asleep, but first you need to make up your mind about your basic approach. There are two main views – it's up to you to decide which you naturally feel comfortable with.

1 *Do you want your baby to learn to get to sleep without you?*
   At bedtime, eight-month-old Jasmine was put to sleep in her cot in the corner of her parents' bedroom. They'd say 'night-night', give her a kiss and tuck her in. She would stare at her mobile above the cot for a while and then call

for her parents for a few minutes. They left the door slightly ajar with the landing light on, so they could keep a watch on her, and after five or ten minutes she would fall asleep on her own. She would sometimes cry in the night, but her parents tried to leave her and most of the time she would fall back to sleep quickly on her own.

2 *Or do you want your baby in bed with you as he falls asleep – both at bedtime and when he wakes in the night?* Leslie and Nick's third child, Luke, never settled easily as a baby. Their older two, Debbie and Mandy, had slept in their parents' bed when they were younger but now chose to sleep in their own beds. Leslie and Nick decided to follow the same pattern and let Luke sleep with them. After a bath and some stories, one parent would stay with Luke at bedtime until he fell asleep. Sometimes this wouldn't take long, while on other nights they had to stay with him for an hour or more. If Luke woke during the evening (before they had gone to bed) they would have to go to be with him. Mostly, though, Leslie and Nick would have some time to themselves in the evening and then join Luke later on.

Of course, only you can decide which of these approaches suits you. Whichever way you choose for coping between three and six months, however, the reality is that, if you want your baby to 'sleep through the night', he needs to learn how to fall asleep, at bedtime and in the middle of the night, without needing you.

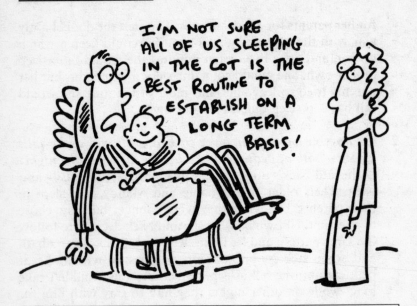

I'M NOT SURE ALL OF US SLEEPING IN THE COT IS THE BEST ROUTINE TO ESTABLISH ON A LONG TERM BASIS!

Top Tip: *Decide where, when and how you really want your baby to sleep, and develop a routine now.*

Reading the signs of sleepiness

Your baby gives you clues when he's tired and needs a rest. Typical signs are:

- not being able to concentrate on anything for long, or

- suddenly becoming more alert;
- being excited, 'hyperactive' and bouncy;
- ear-pulling;
- getting upset easily;
- sucking his fingers;
- rubbing his eyes;
- being grumpy, bad-tempered and miserable around the same time each day.

Become sensitive to your baby's individual signals and keep an eye out for them. Very rarely will a child offer to go to sleep, even if he is tired.

> **Top Tip:** *Learn to read your baby's signals so that you know when he is tired and ready for sleep.*

Daytime sleeps

Babies who aren't sleeping well at night often aren't sleeping well in the daytime either. If at all possible, get into the habit of letting your baby have a daytime sleep in his cot, and the nights will often sort themselves out on their own. Put your baby in his cot at the time he regularly gets tired during the day, as he will find this the easiest time to fall asleep. If you miss the moment and he gets overtired, it will be much harder for him to relax enough to fall asleep.

Top Tip: *If your baby has an established sleep time in the day it will help him learn to sleep well at night.*

The downside of this is that a regular routine can disrupt your social life for a while – but that's all part and parcel of being a parent. Shopping trips, visits from adoring relatives, aerobics sessions (though some of you might have been looking for a good excuse to miss these anyway!) are not as important as seeing that your baby gets the rest he needs. Don't expect him to smile sweetly at the Italian waiter if you're out eating pizza when all he wants is his lunchtime nap.

Fitting daytime sleeps into other siblings' routines

All this is not always easy – especially with the arrival of a second, third or fourth child. An older child has to be at school or football practice, and just at the time the baby would really appreciate being tucked into bed. It will take a fair amount of juggling, but ensuring that your baby gets some uninterrupted daytime sleep is, in reality, an investment for both of you. That said, however, 'some rules were made to be broken'! As long as a well-established regular daytime sleep routine exists there will still be room for a bit of flexibility from time to time.

Getting into a bedtime routine that suits you and your baby

A bedtime routine can also be really helpful in getting your baby to settle. It's a signal to him that bedtime is coming. A typical routine could be having a bath, brushing his teeth (if he's got any!), reading stories, singing songs and having a drink of milk (breast or bottle). However tempting it is to play British Bulldog as bedtime approaches, or to impress him with your hungry lion impersonations, it is rather more effective to create an atmosphere of calm, with low lighting and not too much stimulation. Be as creative as you like, but do yourself a favour and don't create a routine that takes two hours to get through.

> **Top Tip:** Developing a regular bedtime routine helps to give your baby the signal that bedtime isn't far away.

Sleep associations

When he's between four and six months old, your baby will begin to learn to fall asleep by taking into account the familiar cues that are around him. If he then wakes up in the night, he will expect the same cues to be around him in order to go back to sleep again. It's a good idea, therefore, to think about what kind of things your baby associates with sleep. He may have learnt to rely on the smell of the room, his blanket, dummy, teddy and other familiar objects. You might have a musical mobile or sing lullabies that signal sleep time. In many cases, if you've allowed him to, he may also have come to see the presence of at least one of his parents as a prerequisite for falling asleep. Though this is fine to begin with, if you want to sleep through the night it may be better in the longer term to choose a comforter that doesn't rely on your presence.

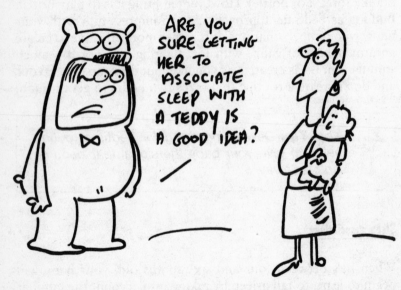

As babies tend to become attached to favourite objects from any point between six and eighteen months, this might be the time to encourage the regular use of a sleep-time comforter. Soft toys or blankets work well, and it'll make life a lot easier for you if the comforter is replaceable, easily transportable and washable.

Dummies can be a help, until they get lost in the bedclothes! Your child is less likely to lose his thumb, so it may prove a better alternative for a baby who really loves to suck.

> **Top Tip:** As he gets older, your baby learns how to fall asleep by taking in the familiar 'cues' that are around him. If he wakes in the night, he'll look for these cues again in order to go back to sleep. This may include you being nearby!

Actions speak louder than words

So much about sleep is really about personality – your baby's (which you won't change or alter however much you'd like to), and yours, as the parent. If your tendency is to scream '*GO TO SLEEP!*' while towering over his cot and turning an unhealthy shade of puce, your baby will think you are either funny or frightening. But one way or the other, it's not going to help him to fall asleep. However irritated you're feeling, do your best to keep as calm and soft in tone as possible. The golden rule is, the calmer you appear the more quickly your baby will calm down and fall asleep.

> **Top Tip:** Even if he's driving you up the wall, the calmer you can appear to be the more quickly your baby will calm down!

If you put him to bed in a darkened room, whisper 'night-night' (not hiss it through gritted teeth) and leave him to go to sleep, he may well cry, but he'll slowly begin to get the idea of what you're expecting him to do. Consistently repeating this little scenario, combined with your maintaining an air of 'I'm incredibly dull and boring to be with at this time of day', will mean he soon learns that there's not much point in calling out for you . . . *'No more entertainment or attention tonight then, huh? I'll just check one more time . . . One last cry to see if I can get any reaction . . . Nope, looks like this is night-time and I may as well go to sleep.'*

What affects sleep in a three- to six-month-old?

Let's look at the commonest reasons that babies of this age have trouble getting themselves back to sleep:

Sucking to sleep

Many babies at this age have become used to falling asleep while sucking – on a bottle, a dummy or Mum's breast. It's one of the most common reasons why babies of this age are restless during the night. When they wake up during the 'light sleep' stage of their sleep cycle, they simply cannot get back to sleep unless they are sucking. If you want your baby to fall asleep on his own without you giving him a dummy or a feed, you have to teach him how.

It's natural to put a sleeping baby quietly in his cot after a feed and tip-toe out of the room with a contented grin on your face. You slump into an armchair, thinking 'Peace at last!' But the problem is, the evening's activity doesn't usually end there. As soon as he reaches the light sleeping stage of his sleep cycle, your baby wakes up – and who does he want to help him go back to sleep? You!

If your baby wakes up at night 'for a feed', but then only has two sucks on the breast or bottle before falling asleep again, you can safely assume that it's not hunger that's woken him up. He just wants to suck as a comforter before he can fall asleep again. Don't blame him, it's not his problem – he won't learn how to fall asleep on his own unless you change this routine.

 Top Tip: *If you want your baby to fall asleep on his own without you giving him a dummy or a feed, you have to teach him how.*

Some parents choose to wait until their child has had his first birthday before trying to change this kind of routine. Others prefer to be a bit stricter earlier on (maybe at six months or so). Either way, don't feel pressurised to do anything you don't want to. There isn't some Big Mother in the sky watching you, taking notes!

But when you are ready, how do you change his sleeping habits? There are a couple of options.

Option 1 The kamikaze option: when he's drowsy at the end of the feed, give him a nudge, waking him slightly as you put him in the cot. If you're lucky he'll open one eye, realise you're putting him in his cot and then fall asleep. To be honest, it's more likely that he will wake up, scream and leave you with the job of spending another half an hour calming him down again! Many mums and dads talk about their baby's in-built 'plumb line' which can sense them being lowered into their cot, triggering a screaming session. The thing to remember, however, is that although in the short term it can be hard going, by putting him in bed awake you're giving him the chance to learn how to fall asleep without you. He'll also begin to get the message that there's nothing frightening about falling asleep.

Option 2 A much less stressful solution can be to make your baby's bedtime feed slightly earlier, say half an hour before usual. This means that by the end of the feed he is ready to sleep but still awake enough to realise what's going on. You might still have some crying to contend with, but if your baby's tired it's unlikely to be too long before he falls asleep.

The next chapter looks in much more detail at seven key ways of helping your child go to sleep. Whichever option you choose, however, you'll find it works best if you begin to make changes with his *daytime* sleeps first, rather than at bedtime or during the night. There is a good reason for this. In the day, your baby will be tired and needing sleep, but you're more likely to be wide-awake and strong-willed. At night it's usually the other way around! Creating good sleep habits for your baby during the day will have a ripple effect over the following weeks. Bedtime settling is likely to become much less complicated once you've cracked his daytime sleep routine.

Dummies

The issue of dummies is a controversial one among parents (and often grandparents). Though they can quickly become a child's – and subsequently the parent's – main comforter, especially in the early months, they can sometimes cause more grief than they've been worth after three to six months.

The problem with a dummy at this age comes when your child relies on it to suck himself to sleep. It's back to those sleep associations again: whether it's bottle-feeding, breast-feeding or dummy-sucking, he'll learn to depend on these being provided in order for him to go to sleep. Of course, using a dummy doesn't require you to be there, but once the dummy falls out, if he can't find it and put it back in his mouth he'll cry out for you to put it back in! Many parents are happy to quickly pop the dummy back in; others would prefer not to get out of bed at all and choose to teach their baby to fall asleep without one. A friend of mine made sure her son had ten dummies in the bed so he always managed to find one eventually! So there are times when a dummy can be really useful and times when they can cause some grief – it's up to you to decide if, or when, to use one.

The same rule applies to dummies as to any other sleep habit: if you're not happy with the situation you find yourself in, try to do something about it sooner rather than later. The longer you leave it, the harder it will be for your baby to learn new ways of getting to sleep.

> **Top Tip:** *The difference between a child who sleeps through the night and one who is up several times lies not in the number of times they are awake, but in their ability to go back to sleep without needing any extra help.*

Wriggling babies

Once your baby starts moving in his cot at night, the advice on sleep positions no longer applies – lying them on their backs is only important when they are too young to be able to move themselves. So don't waste your energies repositioning your baby only to find him back lying on his tummy two minutes later!

Both my children seemed to wriggle for England in their cots at night and woke regularly, feeling cold, sitting on top of their blankets. Most babies have cold hands and feet, but this will not affect their sleep. If, on the other hand, they become cold either on their chests or between the shoulder blades, they will usually wake up and cry.

Using a process of trial and error, my husband Nick and I eventually worked out how many layers of bedclothes our children needed at different times of year. However, for us, night-time fleece babygros (rather than using blankets) have proved an excellent solution for our wriggly babies, and they may do for yours, too.

The first tooth

My six-month-old son was really tetchy and miserable for a few days and I couldn't work out why. Then a friend turned up with a suggestion. Four adults kneeling round the baby, trying to get him to do a roaring lion impression, finally paid off as he opened his mouth wide to reveal a tiny speck of enamel, prompting a huge howl of relief from his mother as she realised he was teething.

In one sense teething is wonderful – you can use it to explain away every bit of bad baby behaviour! In other ways, however, it is murder. Babies can't put into words how it feels to have their gums pierced, but we can all imagine just how unpleasant it is. If you've ever had toothache you will know how impossible it is to fall asleep – especially in the middle of the night – and so it's unsurprising that this particular stage of a baby's development brings with it more than its usual share of howling and broken nights.

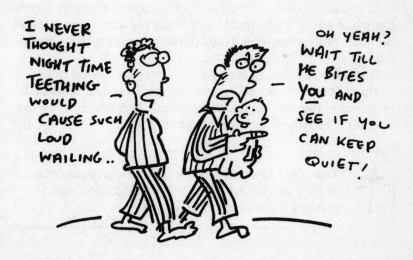

Common signs associated with teething are:

- copious dribbling;
- wanting to chew on everything;
- bright red cheeks which make him look as though he's been on a three-mile jog on a winter morning;
- runny, acidic poo that can burn the skin and cause nappy rash;
- being generally grouchy.

Use baby paracetamol and teething gels according to their instructions to help relieve the pain before bed and in the night. To protect your baby's skin, use Vaseline on his chin and lots of thick barrier cream on his bottom. (One extra point here: if you're using today's modern 'super-dooper' nappies, just stick to the Vaseline on his chin. For these nappies, a barrier cream can make nappy rash worse, as it keeps the acidic poo against the skin and prevents it from passing through the stay-dry lining.)

And to be honest, in terms of his sleeping during bouts of teething, don't expect too much! In many mums' and dads' experience, though, if you know what's keeping them awake at night it somehow seems more manageable.

 Top Tip: Teething's not much fun for your baby or for you, but there are some things you can do to make it easier on both of you.

Weaning on to solid food

This is the age when not only teeth start shooting through, but carrot puree and baby rice as well! Between the ages of four and six months, milk alone won't satisfy your baby's appetite and it's time to start solid food. The good news is that many parents say their nights become more settled once their baby is taking solids. And what's more, as the amount of solid food gradually increases, your baby won't have enough tummy space to put away the same amount of milk. As a result, the milk feeds will get smaller, so be ready for it and don't worry when it happens.

But I'm still hungry!

As we've already said, starting solid food may also produce a change for the better in your baby's night-time sleeping pattern. The more he feeds in the day, the less he will need to feed at night. But if he still wakes and wants to consume a large feed in the night, it's simply not worth trying to delay it by fobbing him off with a drink of water – a hungry baby won't settle until he's fed. If, on the other hand, he's waking simply for two sucks of milk and then falling back to sleep, it's a different story altogether. If he only takes tiny amounts of milk, there's every chance that it's not hunger that's woken him at all. So check to see if he's dirty, very wet, too hot or too cold. It could also be that he's been used to sucking himself to sleep (see pages 54–5). You'll soon know if the reason is boredom or wanting attention because he'll normally stop crying as soon as you go to him.

My daughter used to cry in the night, but as soon as I picked her up she'd just smile at me – the broadest, twinkliest smile she could. The first few nights it happened, I sat there and gazed at her, smiling back. It took about two weeks for the novelty to wear off, by which time I'd decided that these smiling sessions would be far more enjoyable at 8 a.m., instead of 4 a.m.! I started to leave her and, sure enough, she'd begin to cry. Amazingly, however, this burst of bawling would only last for five minutes or so, with her eventually falling back to sleep on her own. Although leaving her was very hard to do at the time, we made sure we had time for our smiling sessions in the morning to make up for it!

This three-to-six-month stage can be an uncertain time for parents, because your baby will be changing his habits so quickly as he develops. His voice and language, the way he sleeps and the way he moves his body are all changing fast. There'll be aspects of the way you care for him which you once felt confident about that will have to change too – and if this baby is your first you'll feel as though you're learning 'on the job'. So don't be too hard on yourself if the nights are still bad at this stage. Once you're certain that your baby doesn't need any milk in the night you can get tougher in persuading him that nights were made for sleeping! Many parents, however, say they don't feel ready to do this until their baby reaches at least six months of age.

It's my night off

If none of the ideas in this book seem to have worked so far, and if you have a partner, take it in turns to be on duty. That way you can at least have every other night off, sleeping somewhere else if you've got space, so that at least one of you gets some sleep to help you face the next morning. When you feel more rested you may feel better prepared to give the ideas another go.

Returning to work

Now may also be the time, if you've taken maternity leave, when you need to return to work. In many ways, the pressure is on for your child to sleep well if you are going back to work full time. Sometimes this pressure can mean that you compromise what you do at night because you're just grateful to get any amount of sleep. Some parents, especially those who work long hours and don't get to spend much time with their baby, find their baby's wakeful times in the night a secret delight, giving them a chance to be alone together. Apart from making sure that you decide on a plan and then stick to it, there's really no across-the-board advice which will fit every situation. Often it will come down to finding an arrangement that you feel will suit you best and then working hard to make it happen. Here are some tips which may help:

- Try to decide where and how you want your child to sleep *before* you go back to work.
- Recognise and talk about the tension that returning to work can bring – spending your nights worrying about how you're going to cope at work tomorrow will not help anyone.

- Some parents who are experiencing very disrupted nights (and whose jobs allow them to) choose to tackle the problem head on. They take a block of holiday at once (say, a week), but stay at home and toughen their resolve for sorting out the sleep routines during this time. Solving your child's sleep problems might not be everyone's idea of a great holiday, but you can always spend fantastic days together with your child and you won't have the worry of how you're going to cope at work the next day.
- If the disruptions at night are taking their toll on your work, talk to your employer about it – they may be more flexible than you had imagined. Let them know the impact it's having at the moment, but make sure they know that you're in the process of sorting things out (and that you're reading this great book that's going to help you . . .).

 Top Tip: *If you're returning to work, think about the sleep issues you're likely to face before you do so.*

'Can I phone a friend, please?'

Following an early run of enthusiastic offers of help, by the time your baby is three to six months old these may be beginning to dry up a little. It's important to remember that looking after yourself and finding enough time out from caring for your child is vital, especially if he isn't sleeping well. And if you're looking after children on your own it's even more important. There is absolutely no shame or blame in having a baby who is struggling to get to grips with sleeping – nearly all parents face problems in this department at one time or another. So don't be reluctant to ask your friends and family for the help to continue. If you don't make sure people know you're finding things tough, they may assume that you are coping fine and don't need their help any more.

Top Tip: If your baby is between three and six months old, you're reading this book at the best possible moment. Now is the time to begin thinking about how and where you want your family to sleep. Learn to read your baby's tiredness cues and get into good habits for the future. This is your mission, should you choose to accept it – but it's not a mission impossible!

Getting Some Sleep: The Top Seven Options on the Road to Freedom

If you want to change your baby's sleep habits, this chapter describes seven possible ways to go about doing it. Though I've just explained that between three and six months is the ideal moment to change a baby's sleeping habits, if your child is already older . . . relax! All the options here can work for babies from three months old to children of seven years and beyond. However, some are better suited to particular ages than others, so look out for the options that will best suit you and your child.

First things first

I know that it's incredibly tempting to race on into this chapter to discover (I hope) the secret to unlocking sleep-filled nights for ever. But first things first. Before trying to change your baby's sleeping habits, it may be wise first to have a look at what you might already be doing that could be working against your child sleeping well.

If you've read all the earlier chapters of this book, there have probably been things that have already struck you as patterns or habits you would like to change. As we've already seen, it's all too easy for mums and dads to slip into routines that aren't entirely helpful when it comes to encouraging healthy sleep patterns for their children. So a quick honest look at what's already going on could make all the difference.

> **Top Tip:** Before trying to change your baby's sleeping habits, take an honest look at what you are already doing – and what you're prepared to do to encourage change.

Sleep diaries

I'm a great fan of lists and writing things down – mainly because my memory is the size of a Malteser. By writing down what happens at night you can build up an accurate picture of what is actually going on, rather than blearily trying to remember the events of the night before. Added to that, when you're desperate to get some sleep it's common to try a variety of methods, which means that a sleep diary can help pinpoint which ones worked.

It doesn't matter what the diary looks like, but it's useful to note the following facts:

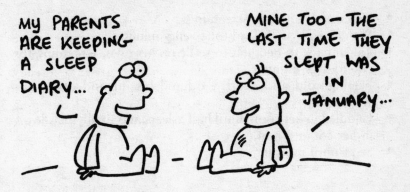

- the time your baby wakes in the morning;
- her mood on waking;
- the time of nap/s in the day;
- the time she goes to bed in the evening;
- the time she goes to sleep at bedtime;
- the time she wakes in the night;
- what you do when she wakes;
- the time/s she goes to sleep again.

Here's an example, the sleep diary of sixteen-month-old Courteney:

Wednesday
- Woke at 7 a.m., grumpy.
- Usual two-hour nap after lunch.
- Bedtime at 7.30 p.m. with cup of warm milk.
- Cried for ten minutes, then fell asleep.

- Woke at 1.15 a.m., screaming.
- Watched TV with Dad for twenty minutes.
- Taken back to bed, left to settle on her own, screaming for twenty-five minutes.
- Feeling cold and snuffly, offered biscuit and drink but wasn't thirsty.
- Cuddled in her room until half asleep, and finally put down in her cot at 3 a.m.
- Slept until morning.

Thursday
- Woke at 8 a.m.
- Usual two-hour sleep after lunch.
- In bed by 7 p.m., settled by 7.05 p.m.
- Woke screaming at 4 a.m.
- Left to settle on her own; after ten minutes went back to sleep.
- Slept until 6.45 a.m.

Friday
- Everyone woken up by someone at the door, 7.15 a.m.
- Courteney tired by 11 a.m. but managed to give her her lunch early.
- Fell asleep as soon as I put her in bed, at 11.45 a.m.
- Slept until 2.30 p.m.
- Busy afternoon, lots of friends round.
- In bed by 8 p.m., really tired.
- Slept through until 8 a.m.!

Hopefully, your sleep diary will help you to pinpoint things that work (or don't), and also provide a bit of much needed encouragement as you see things are beginning to improve. If you need some extra help in working out an action plan from your diary, ask a friend you trust, another parent you respect or your health visitor to take a look at it. They will have a fresh pair of eyes and may be able to tease out the problems.

Top Tip: *Sleep diaries can help you to tease out the issues that are affecting your child's sleep and help you decide what to do about them.*

That's when good neighbours become good friends

It's worth letting your neighbours know when you plan to change sleeping routines and warn them that there might be a week of crying in the night. If your walls are very thin, they may be more supportive if you ask them if there is any particular day or week to avoid when tackling the problem. Although there's always that feeling that someone may call Social Services, most neighbours will, of course, be keen to help you get the problem sorted out so that everyone concerned can get a good night's sleep.

The seven steps to sleep-filled nights

So here they are – the top seven options to get you and your child on the road to a better night's sleep.

1 Wait till they grow out of it

This involves doing nothing different and just sitting it out. This does work for some parents – it's just a matter of whether your nerve holds. You can recite to yourself 'it's only a passing phase . . . it's only a passing phase', if that helps pass the time. However, sitting it out won't speed up the process of getting a good night's sleep, so if you're getting really heated about things it's worth considering taking a more direct approach to change your situation.

2 All in bed together

This is a popular option with parents when they've given up trying to persuade their child to fall asleep on her own. It's easy to see why:

- Children, especially babies, often sleep well when they are near their parents.
- There is none of the crying, screaming and head-banging which is often involved in getting them to sleep in their own cots.
- Regardless of how you feed your child, there are fewer disturbances if you're all in bed together. If Mum is breast-feeding, neither parent need even get out of bed!

If you decide to share the bed with your child, make sure your partner feels as happy as you do about the arrangement. If you have different views, it's really important that you listen to each other and try to work out a compromise. Obviously, being consistent in your approach to bedtime routines and night-time sleeping will help your child settle much more quickly than if you opt for a different method each night.

You won't need me to tell you to get as big a bed as you can. In fact, I know of one family who liked their space so much that they arranged two double futon mattresses lying together on the floor! As a big family, they found it gave them extra flexibility and comfort and no one was left hanging off the edge of the bed. The decision to do something like this is better made early on, so you can really *sleep* together as a family – in comfort, not agony!

Some of the disadvantages to bed-sharing are that

- Breast-feeding babies may be tempted to wake up and feed much more frequently than they would if a full breast of milk wasn't two inches from their nose.
- Your child may be more wriggly than an escapologist or prefer lying on top of you or across the width of the bed. Great for her, but a disaster for you – she may 'sleep like a baby' but you may not!
- You may feel as though you never get a break from your child.

The Department of Health advises against bed-sharing if either you or your partner smoke, have taken drugs which make you drowsy (whether medical or recreational, and including alcohol) or if you're very tired, especially with a young baby. Even if none of the above applies, and despite the research being inconclusive into whether bed-sharing has any impact on a baby's health (particularly with regard to cot death), it still errs on the side of caution. In fact, the DoH goes so far as to recommend that, should you choose to comfort your baby in bed, you still put her back in her own cot to actually *sleep*. (See Chapter 4 for more details.)

3 The Controlled Crying option

This is the first of three options (numbers 3, 4 and 5 in this list) which all involve letting your child fall asleep without receiving any of your attention (cuddles, drinks, songs, stories, etc.). The differences between the techniques are subtle (blink and you might miss them), but basically they are differentiated by how often you go back to your child once she has been put to bed. With Controlled Crying, you lengthen the gap between your visits; with the Elastic Band method, you stay in her room until she falls asleep, and in the case of the Checking method you go in regularly every five minutes.

 Top Tip: *Controlled Crying is all about helping your child to fall asleep, but with minimum intervention from you.*

Controlled Crying is a common choice for many parents of younger children because it is very effective when mums and dads carry it out consistently.

After your bedtime routine:

- Say, 'Go to sleep now, night-night,' and leave the room – even if she is crying and calling for you.
- If you are particularly sensitive to her cry, go in after one minute. If you feel stronger and are able to, leave her alone for two to three minutes.
- Go to reassure her – but try to be as boring as possible. Whatever you do don't lift her up!
- Leave fairly promptly, saying, 'Go to sleep now, night-night.'
- Repeat the process again, lengthening the gap between your visits by five minutes. Don't leave her any longer than twenty minutes at any one go.
- Keep going with the routine at a pace that you can manage.

If your baby is a 'good screamer' and has been blessed with an effective pair of lungs, this method can be hard going at first, but it actually has a very good track record of success. If she wakes in the night you should go through exactly the same process again. If it's going to work, it'll happen within a week or so.

Key points to remember are:

- Try and build up the length of time you leave your baby as soon as you can.
- Never leave your baby to cry on her own for more than twenty minutes at a time.
- Try to give her as little eye contact or attention as possible when you go to her. Make your visit as boring and mundane

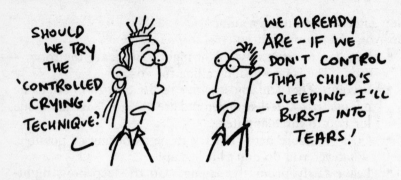

as possible. Resist all temptation to pick her up and cuddle her!

- Be consistent night after night.

4 The Elastic Band option

This is a particularly good method if you've tried leaving your child before, but have been exhausted by her ability to cry for particularly long periods of time (some children have been known to hit three-hour stretches!). It works, especially for parents and children who've found Controlled Crying too traumatic, because you offer your child reassurance by staying with her but give no other incentive to stay awake.

It's a method which comes across as hard work for parents, but it has a good success rate and can be gentler for babies and parents alike. Many parents and health visitors swear by it.

Nothing to do with twanging rubber bands to the tune of 'Rock-a-bye baby', the Elastic Band method works by teaching your child to fall asleep on her own. All the time, however, you stay in her room until she falls asleep, making sure that she can see you and knows that you are still nearby for her.

 Top Tip: *The Elastic Band method shows your child that, although you're still nearby if she needs you, she can fall asleep on her own.*

The Elastic Band method is based on a number of key actions:

- As with every option, you need to be motivated before you begin.
- Whatever you do to aid her going to sleep in her bedroom should only be as an extension of a firmly established bedtime routine. You should resist the temptation to bring your child back into the living area of your home once she's had a bath or bedtime story. Lights and noise levels should also be kept low. If you don't, there's little chance of the 'no more entertainment now because it's bedtime' message getting through!
- You must always stay within your child's line of vision and must not leave the room.
- You should never make eye contact with your child once you've put her in her cot. This is vitally important. Experts on this method of sleep training suggest, for those parents who find it difficult avoiding eye contact, that focusing on another part of the child's body (i.e. her shoulder or her feet) can help.
- You begin by placing her in her cot, asking her to stay lying

there, and then move slowly backwards and forwards between her cot and her bedroom door. This is the 'elastic band' bit – you leave her cot, then return again, perhaps only thirty seconds later.

- You should try to keep interaction with her to the absolute minimum until she falls asleep.
- But if your child is upset, you *can* reassure her with your touch – hold her hand and even hug her – as long as her bottom stays touching the cot. Again, though, whatever you do, don't look at her!
- You can only leave the room once she is asleep.

Having read the last eight points, you may find it difficult to visualise yourself wandering backwards and forwards between her cot and the door for hours on end (especially if your child's room is really tiny), but it really does work. And you don't have to *just* walk backwards and forwards between her cot and the door; you could take the opportunity to tidy up her clothes, pack away her toys – potter around. The point is, by being there you build up a trust between you and your child that increases her confidence to fall asleep without the fear of being left alone.

If your child is very distressed, and providing you don't look at her or pick her up, go to her quickly to reassure her. Lower the cot side, kneel down beside it and hold her if you wish. By doing this you're teaching her that you'll come to comfort her, but it's also bedtime and bed is where she is going to stay. Once the crying has stopped, put the cot side back up and carry on walking from the door to the cot. Return to keeping your contact with her as minimal as possible and stay in the room until she has fallen asleep.

When she wakes in the night you do the same thing all over again – walking up and down from her side to the door and back, touch her as long as she's lying down, and stay with her until she's fallen asleep. Do this every time she wakes.

Your child might be stunned and angry at your refusal to pick her up or give her any attention, but she won't cry due to fear of being left. Mums and dads who've tried this technique say that their child's reaction is much less distressing, and that it is easier to put into practice because they know their child is not scared, just cross. For most of them it's a case of 'Hey, she's not the only one who's cross around here!'

 Top Tip: *Avoiding eye contact with your child is a vital ingredient for success with the Elastic Band method, but you can reassure her with your touch at any time.*

For some, the first night can be the worst – you may have to stay with your child for up to an hour and a half. For others, the novelty of a new bedtime routine makes it the easiest night, with their child falling asleep in ten or twenty minutes. If she has found the first night easy, your child may want to revert to her old ways on the second night, and as a result it can be the hardest. By the fourth or fifth night, you'll be seeing progress and will begin to feel in control again.

You may find it helpful to keep a note of how long it takes before she falls asleep, so that you can see how she is improving. As I said at the outset, you will need to be motivated to keep

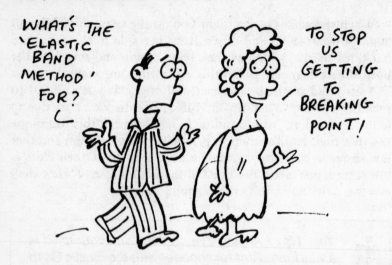

going throughout the whole week – and believe me, it's a real encouragement to see changes happening before your eyes. Best of all, you will eventually have the greater reward of a lifetime of sleep ahead of you!

However, if you would rather not stay in your child's room at all, Option 5 might be for you. It's known as 'Checking'.

5 The Checking option

I'll come clean: we used this option with our children, and still need to from time to time, especially after illness and holidays. It is a good method for all ages, from babies of three months to school-age children. This method is similar in concept to the Elastic Band approach because it reassures your child that you are nearby and helps you to know that your child is safe and well. The main difference, however, is that you don't stay in your child's room.

Unlike flat-pack storage units from your local DIY store, the Checking method has easy-to-follow instructions! After saying, 'It's bedtime, go to sleep now,' you leave your child to go to sleep. If you have a young baby, wait for two minutes before going back to her and repeat the same 'night-night' message. For older children, five-minute intervals work better. Whichever you choose, simply pop in again after the same time interval (no more, no less), recite your bedtime message like a broken record, and leave again. Repeat this routine until she falls asleep. You'll need a watch to time each two- or five-minute interval.

 Top Tip: When using the Checking method, maintaining the same interval between visits to your child is crucial.

Many parents who've tried this say the five minutes goes so quickly that they've barely left their child before they are due to go and reassure them again. They don't have time to pace up and down the landing feeling like wretched evil parents. Knowing that they are going back to their child so soon makes them feel less guilty and, as a result, more confident when they do return to her. This in turn helps their child feel more confident about being left to go to sleep.

The golden rule, again, is be as boring as possible and don't pick your child up. And you must stick to your plan like super-glue – don't give in after a few nights or you'll have wasted all your hard work! It would be like that time when you got fed up in the post office queue and left, not realising that, if you'd only waited a minute more, you would have reached the front.

After three to six nights most children give in and sleep well, having learnt that, although Mum or Dad always comes back, they don't pay them any nice attention. Their crying simply isn't bringing the same rewards as before.

However, for a small number of children this method doesn't work at all. Each time you go in, the child will become more and more hysterical. So if you've tried this for an hour or more to no effect, try either the Elastic Band method or Option 6, the Softly Softly approach.

6 The Softly Softly approach

This is another gentle method, and will take perhaps months rather than weeks to achieve your ultimate goal. However, despite the long time-scale it can seem much kinder to everyone and is particularly good for older children. It works by letting your child gradually learn to fall asleep in small manageable steps. This is a really good method if you have tried other ways without success or if your toddler has always slept badly.

However tempting it may be to try to solve all the issues in one night, people who succeed in managing sleep difficulties do so because they don't bite off more than they, or their child, can chew in one go. The key with the Softly Softly approach is to divide the job into small steps and make each step last at least a week (more if necessary) before moving on to the next one. It's a slow but sure way of changing behaviour, and it's very successful if you stick to your plan.

Top Tip: *The Softly Softly approach works by you taking lots and lots of small manageable steps.*

Take Patrick as an example:

Eight-month-old Patrick used to have five bottles of milk (of between four and eight ounces each) and three solid meals during the day. He still woke for a bottle in the night, around 4 a.m., but would take only two or three ounces. Sometimes he would fall asleep before he'd finished the bottle. Neil, his dad, had tried to let him cry it out – refusing him a bottle – but Patrick would get hysterical and it would then take a good hour to settle him again, by which time it would be nearly morning. Neil decided on the Softly Softly approach in order to stop him having the night-time bottle. He decided he would gradually reduce the amount of milk he gave Patrick and begin to offer water instead.

During the first week Neil offered Patrick a three-ounce bottle of milk. In the second week, Neil offered him two ounces of formula milk. Throughout the third week he offered one ounce of milk. For the fourth week, he offered only water, which Patrick rejected, preferring instead to settle without any drink at all in the night. This established his sleeping routine for the future. Neil made sure that Patrick had the chance to feed well during the day on solids, so that there was no need for him to feed at night.

The whole process took Neil four weeks and resulted in a

happier baby and an even happier dad! The Softly Softly approach is an especially good method for toddlers and school-children, as it gently breaks ingrained habits. For an example of this method working for an older child sharing her parent's bed, read Annie's story on pages 88–9.

> **Top Tip:** It may take longer to reach your goal, but the Softly Softly approach is particularly good for older children, or for changing habits that have been around for a while.

7 Drugs

There are medicines (which only your GP can prescribe for your child) that can provide you with a much needed short-term break if you're in real trouble with your child's sleeping patterns. Things to bear in mind are:

- These prescribed drugs must only be used under medical supervision.
- They can give you a chance to catch up on sleep so you can get enough energy to then choose one of the other options above.
- But medicines are only a temporary measure because they take away the chance for your child to learn to fall asleep on her own and simply sedate her.
- Some medicines have side-effects which themselves can be counter-productive – to be as prepared as possible, always ask your doctor about possible side-effects.

- If you don't use any other method of changing your child's sleep pattern while using medicines, the causes of the problem will be left untackled and so the problems will be likely to continue.

The choice is yours

So there you have it – the top seven options. I hope you find one which works for you. Whichever you choose, though, remember the two golden rules:

1 Before you put your child to bed, go through your mental checklist to make sure that she is well, fed and comfortable.
2 Once you've decided which option you're going to try, decide how you're going to play it and *stick to it*. Babies need simple rules that stay the same, night after night, in order to give them a chance to learn to change their habits.

If you choose to plump for the Controlled Crying, Checking, Elastic Band or Softly, Softly methods and want your efforts to really pay off, there are four extra pointers that will further heighten your chances of success:

- Ask anyone else who puts your baby to bed, i.e. babysitters, to follow the same routines.
- If your child shares a bedroom with a brother or sister, start your new routine on a Friday night or in the school holidays. This means that whoever shares the room will

have a better chance of getting a lie-in if they are disturbed during the night.

- Try to plan plenty of time to recover and catch up on lost sleep. Keep your weekends or time off free from visitors (unless they've come to baby-sit while you have a nap).
- Choose your time to begin. If it's a particularly busy time at home or work, or if you're about to go on holiday or move home, it may be a better idea to save it until things calm down a bit.

Once your child is over six months old, the chances are that she will learn to fall asleep using any of the first six options (saving you the stress of having to resort to Option 7). But for the time being, think about which feels most suitable for your family and go for it.

Good luck, and here's to sleep-filled nights!

 Top Tip: *Once you've decided which option you're going to try, decide how you're going to play it and stick to it.*

Six to Twelve Months

Assuming your baby has read all the parenting manuals, he should by now be sleeping through the night! But the fact that you're reading this chapter of this book implies that maybe he isn't.

Between six months and a year, babies need roughly fifteen hours' sleep in every twenty-four, including two to four hours during the day. However, your friend's baby of the same age is sleeping through now, while yours still insists on tripping the light fantastic well into the early hours. Don't panic . . . both you and your child are normal. Research shows that one in every five children aged nine months still has settling difficulties, and two in five wake regularly during the night. Listening to your baby's screams has been compared to having a pneumatic drill in your head and so, ten to twelve months after the birth, it's not surprising that parents of babies who still aren't sleeping well have had enough and want to change.

If you've skipped straight to this page (because your child is between six and twelve months old), go back and take a quick look at Chapter 6, which lists the top seven options for changing your child's night-time behaviour. Many parents have found these provide the solution to their problems – normally without too many tears.

But there's more good news, because at this stage there are other things you can do to make things better.

Some of the basic principles covered in earlier chapters are almost certainly worth sticking to for your six-to-twelve-month old, too. For instance, deciding where and when you want your baby to sleep, agreeing how and when to start teaching him good sleeping habits, and learning how to read his tiredness cues will all play a considerable part in leading to sleep-filled nights for you and your baby. However, in cases where children aged between six and twelve months continue to suffer from disturbed sleep, the cause can often be related to other factors. Your sleepless nights could be down to any of the following:

- Inappropriate boundaries
- Daytime sleeps
- Bedtime routines
- Craving attention
- Crying
- Night-time breast-feeding

Inappropriate boundaries

Karen lives in a one-bedroom flat with Annie, her two-year-old daughter. Annie, who is asthmatic, sleeps in a cot next to her mum's double bed. Annie would only fall asleep if she was holding her mum in the big bed. As she eventually fell asleep, Karen would loosen Annie's grip, gently move her over to her cot (which is level with the mattress) and tip-toe out of the room. It usually took her an hour and a half to settle her. But in the night, when Annie woke up she would head straight back into her mum's bed.

Karen was very keen to get Annie to learn to fall asleep on her own in her own cot. The first time she tried leaving her in the cot, Annie suffered an asthma attack because she got so upset. Because of this Karen realised that leaving Annie alone even for a few minutes was too big a step for her to take, so with the help of her health visitor she set herself a smaller, more achievable target. Karen started to encourage Annie to fall asleep lying next to her on the bed but without hugging. Each time Annie went to hug her mum, Karen would lay her back on her side, saying, 'Time to go to sleep now.'

After a week, Annie was falling asleep without hugging, and so Karen felt confident enough to take the next step. This involved her lying further away from Annie, so they weren't touching but were still lying on the bed with each other. The following week Annie lay in her cot while Karen stayed on the bed. The next step was for Karen to sit by the door, then in the doorway, and then outside the door, and she did each of these for seven nights.

The whole process took about four months from beginning to end. Annie now falls asleep on her own without any trouble.

There's an old saying which goes 'Good fences make good neighbours' – and the more you think about it, the more it makes sense. Helpful boundaries bring harmony and stability – you know where you stand and the limits of what you can and cannot do. Correct boundaries make you feel secure.

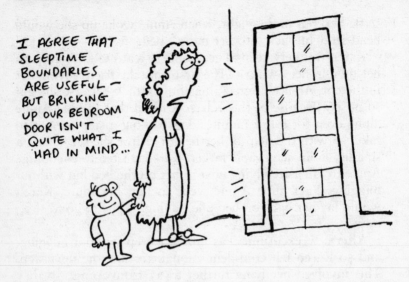

Imagine, for a moment, that you are blindfolded and are left in a room you have never been in before. You don't know how big the room is and you're not sure if there's anything in it. With your arms outstretched, you search for the walls. You knock into something solid which might be a wall. It feels flat and hard so you push it. It wobbles slightly, so you push harder. When it starts to tip over you realise it's not a wall at all, but it may be a cupboard instead. So you carry on searching, knowing that only when you eventually find the walls will you be able to get your bearings about how big the room is and where you are within it. And until that point, the truth is that you'll probably find the whole experience quite unsettling.

Ask almost any parent about the importance of setting boundaries and they will happily agree just how important they are. Setting appropriate boundaries to encourage healthy sleep patterns is no different. Of course, there's another old saying which points out that 'rules are there to be broken', so I guarantee that, as you try to introduce or establish new boundaries, your baby will push to see how firmly you intend to apply them. The question then is, will you wobble like the cupboard or stand immovable like the wall? Your child will test you to see if you mean what you say, but will also feel more secure if you are consistent in how you respond.

> **Top Tip:** Setting boundaries for your child's sleep pattern is a vital ingredient of ensuring that you all get a good night's sleep.

Decide on a routine that you know you can achieve, even if the steps are tiny and very slow at first. If you can succeed in being consistent in applying these small changes, it won't be long before you can speed things up a bit. Nothing succeeds like a bit of success, and small consistent changes will help you to feel on top of things at last. Even better, your baby will sense your attitude is changing. Once he gets wind of your confidence he's likely to follow suit within four to six days.

Daytime sleeps

Although they get in the way of other commitments and, dare I mention, your social life (if you've got the time and energy to have one in the first place!), I'm a firm believer in daytime sleeps. Admittedly, at this age some babies don't need as much sleep, but show me a baby with really bad nights and I'll happily bet £100 he's not sleeping enough during the day. By bedtime, he will be so overtired that there will be very little chance of him settling quickly or easily.

If you are able to base yourself at home, routine and regular daytime sleeps can be a real lifesaver – and, at the same time, your chance to have some time off. If not, it's just a case of trying to find a balance that works for you. For example, it might mean you putting your baby to sleep in his cot at a regular time on the days you can, but for the rest of the week him having to sleep when and wherever he gets the chance.

Top Tip: *Good daytime sleep often helps a child to sleep well at night.*

The timing of daytime sleeps will change as your baby gets older, so if you're unsure about when to put him down in the day, look out for those tell-tale clues that tell you he is tired, and work from there. If he's irritable, miserable, less able to concentrate or rubbing his eyes, chances are he would benefit from a nap. Additionally, try to make sure that he is really physically and mentally stimulated in the day, and avoid daytime sleeps later in the afternoon if you think they make him too perky in the evenings.

Bedtime routines

In the same way as with even younger children, a bedtime routine is valuable because it sends a signal to your baby that bedtime is on its way and coming soon. Once he's picked up the cues he will start to get used to the idea of going to bed. He's much more likely to settle well in his cot if he's had this time to wind down and adjust to the end of his day.

Adults also have bedtime routines. We subconsciously create ways which help us to unwind before bed – finding out what the weather's going to be like tomorrow, having a night-cap or watching a late-night TV programme. My bedtime routine (it's one of my more endearing traits!) is to write lists of all the jobs I need to remember for tomorrow. Only then can I begin to doze off.

Top Tip: *Both adults and children have their bedtime routines. The important thing is to develop one for your child that helps him wind down, ready for sleep.*

You're not going to leave me, are you?

Some babies at this age can begin to show signs of being frightened at being left alone to go to sleep. Babies aren't the only ones – leaving your child to go to sleep can be difficult for parents too! If *you're* looking anxious and unsure as you put your child in the cot, he'll think that something horrible is about

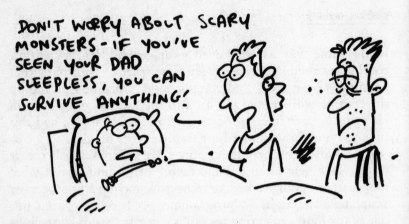

to happen. If you look calm and confident, he's more likely to be relaxed. He'll quickly learn that falling asleep alone doesn't need to be frightening, because he's guided by you. If you find it difficult to leave your child, here are some ideas to try:

- Once your child is in bed, talk about what you have enjoyed together that day and your plans for tomorrow. As you leave your child to go to sleep, you both have in mind nice thoughts of your time together and the anticipation of the fun you'll have together tomorrow.
- Do your best to appear confident, as it will help enormously – bluffing seems to be a skill you need quite a lot in child-rearing, so here's your chance for some hands-on practice!
- When your child finally falls asleep, spend some time watching him and enjoy looking at him. Notice the sound and speed of his breathing; keep a picture in your mind of how he looks when he is relaxed.

- For whatever reason, if you still find leaving your child almost impossible, try the Elastic Band method described in Chapter 6. With this method you don't leave your child's room until he is asleep, so the heartache of leaving him is avoided. You are always within his line of vision, but you avoid giving him any attention.

 Top Tip: *The more relaxed and confident you appear to be when leaving your baby, the more relaxed he will be at being left.*

Teddies and other comforts

Many babies from six months old find reassurance in a 'comforter' which can become a great asset in helping them to fall asleep.

You may feel just a little insulted when you realise that you can be replaced by a scruffy teddy or a piece of smelly torn blanket, but children can gain great comfort from having something to hold at night instead of you. A favourite toy or some other object can help them feel less alone and so aid their falling asleep. In fact, some children grow to love their comforter so much that they become almost inseparable from it.

Three-year-old Elliot would only sleep if his bed was covered in toys. His parents tried to get him to sleep with one or two, but every night he'd put them all back before he'd go to sleep. He then developed a fascination for his parents' vacuum cleaner, so to stop him always trying to play with the real one they bought his own toy 'upright'. However, Elliot then insisted that the Hoover came to bed with him, too, and he fell sound asleep every night hugging it!

Other forms of comfort that children often discover themselves are hair-twiddling and thumb-sucking. These are great comforters, as they can't be broken or lost or left at a friend's house twenty miles away!

Top Tip: *When you put your child to sleep, let him hold a 'comforter' – a favourite teddy, a blanket or even his own toy Hoover!*

Craving attention

Any night-time attention from Mum or Dad is a bonus for your baby. Even if you've gone green and smoke is coming out of both ears, for your baby it's better than nothing. Young babies have many ways of ensuring that they get their parents' full attention.

When she was twelve months old, Sam started to be sick, putting her fingers down her throat, when her dad put her in her cot for an afternoon sleep. At first her parents were shocked and rushed into her room with worried-looking faces, lots of eye contact and new sheets. Sam was delighted – so much so that she continued to do it, until her parents realised (by watching her through the crack of the door) that she was deliberately making herself sick and stopped giving her the attention. At first it was hard for them to leave her with vomit on her sheets, but within a couple of days Sam realised her behaviour wasn't getting the attention that she was after. So she rapidly stopped doing it altogether, choosing instead to fall asleep after five or ten minutes' crying.

Another sure-fire-winner attention-seeker is learning to pull yourself upright on to the cot bars. Babies often try this before they've mastered how to drop back down again, and so they yell for help. You rush to him wondering what on earth has happened. You help him down, only for him to pull himself up again. You don't want to leave him stuck standing up, so you stay. And there you are, hanging around feeling that you can't leave, while all the time your little cherub is revelling in your undivided attention. Brilliant!

Instead, choosing to follow the Checking method (pages 79–81) means that you can leave him, knowing that you'll be back in five minutes and no real harm can be done in that time – and your child's boredom may curtail the number of repetitions you have to deal with!

Crying

By six months, most babies have moved on from the 'crying all day' stage. Their cry feels less overwhelming than in the early days, often due to the fact that parents have become more adept at identifying a reason for it. If your baby is still irritable at night, it may be worth discussing this with your health visitor, but it's also very good to remind yourself that crying at bedtime or in the night can very often be a great idea as a way of getting your attention.

It doesn't take all that long for your baby to learn that, when he cries, you come to find out what's wrong. Unsurprisingly, this often encourages him to carry on crying long after your attention is really needed, because he likes your company! Only you can know for sure when this is happening, but when it does it really is crunch time. How you react now will set the pattern for the future, so take time (in the cold light of day) to assess whether you may be doing anything in response to your baby's crying which might give him even more incentive to cry.

Night-time breast-feeding

By six months, most babies are eating enough solids and milk during the day to prevent them from needing a feed in the night. A small number of babies – including those that have been born prematurely – will still need a feed at this age, but most will be feeding for comfort and out of habit rather than because of hunger.

At this stage a common difficulty arises with breast-feeding babies who sleep in or near their parents' bed. Because the milk supply is still constantly available, what was once (at around eight weeks) a major contributor to sleep-filled nights for parents is now the exact opposite! Even though he isn't hungry, he'll nuzzle up to Mum and suck just because she's there. This might not be a problem to you if your sleep is not being terribly disturbed (and your partner can of course be completely oblivious to the problem!), but many mums feel that, by the second half of their child's first year, they've had enough of being woken up in the night – especially when there's really no need.

You don't have to evict your baby from your bed or give up breast-feeding to tackle this situation – the key is to let the baby learn to fall asleep on his own without sucking on the breast. It's easier to start this during the day, when he's more tired than you. Feed him five or ten minutes earlier than usual to prevent him from being so tired at the end of the feed. Then, as you put him in his cot, he will still be aware of his surroundings but drowsy enough to go to sleep. If you can maintain this pattern for daytime sleeps and also at bedtime, you'll find over the next few days that he's less reliant on the need to suck in order to get himself back to sleep at night.

Of course, every baby is different. So if, for any reason, this doesn't work, why not try one of the following options:

- Push your bed up against a wall. Once you've made sure that there are no gaps for your baby to fall down, that the wall is not too cold (if it's an outside wall) or too hot (e.g. next to a radiator), let Dad sleep in the middle with your baby next to the wall. If your bed has castors, you should also make sure that it cannot move away from the wall during the night.
- Move the baby to a cot in your room, or into another room if it's an option.
- Get Dad to offer the baby a cup or feeder-beaker of water when he wakes up. If you manage to combine this with getting him to sleep without sucking milk, within a few

days he will begin to feel that the water is not worth the bother of waking up for.

Crawling towards trouble

There's no time like the present to start tackling sleep habits you don't want to see continue. Now may be the time you decide to teach your baby to sleep in his own cot rather than in your bed, or when you start to cut down (or stop) feeding your baby in the night. Try to stand back from your situation a little and talk it through with someone you trust. You may find that keeping a sleep diary really helps you to see the wood for the trees (see pages 68–70).

One final thing. Don't forget that, if you want your baby to learn how to fall back to sleep on his own in the night, you shouldn't do anything at bedtime that you're not prepared to do in the middle of the night. You'll also have much more success if you help him learn to fall asleep on his own in the daytime first. After that, you can move on to sorting out his night-time antics!

 Top Tip: *Teach him to fall asleep in the daytime first – you'll have more energy to make it happen than at night!*

Soon he'll be taking his first steps, as well as sleeping through the night.

One to Two Years

So at last you've celebrated your baby's first birthday (a friend of mine who has four children tells me that, each time, she has felt that it's more a celebration of her own survival than of her child's birthday!). As with all first birthdays, your child is likely to have spent a fantastic day playing with the box her present came in, while the present itself has remained untouched. And, for you, the fact that your daughter is entering her second year presents an excellent opportunity to take a step back and review your situation. Are you happy with how things are turning out as far as her sleeping is concerned? Is your partner happy? Is your baby happy?

Most children in their second year will sleep between eleven and fifteen hours in every twenty-four, having one to three of those hours in the daytime. You'll probably also be reassured to hear that research shows that one in every five one-year-olds still wakes regularly in the night. Yours isn't the only one! On the other hand, though, if your child is nearly two and you haven't slept through the night once since her birth, you might just be beginning to go round the bend.

This is a fine mess you've got me into, Stanley!

It's perfectly natural for parents of children this age who are not sleeping well during the night to feel they've had enough of being available twenty-four hours a day, desperately needing some proper sleep themselves. Enough is enough, they think. Unfortunately, all this becomes a bit of a vicious circle – you feel so tired and listless that you've no energy to think about alternative and more effective ways of getting your child to sleep, and they wear you out even further. Surely only a miracle will now stop your child waking up in the middle of the night? You feel that you are in a situation which you didn't choose, don't want, but can't find a way out of.

Take heart – helping a two-year-old child to fall asleep at night can be a lot easier than attempting the same thing for a baby. For a start, communication between you both is much more efficient – she is now able to really understand what you are saying to her and is probably beginning to talk. So, for instance, if she is feeling ill or angry she'll certainly let you know. One pitfall, however, is that if her speech is well developed you may unwittingly find yourself in a debate about the merits of bedtime!

 Top Tip: *Never ask an eighteen-month-old if she's ready for bed. One of the first words a baby learns quickly is 'NO'!*

Common issues that affect sleep at between one and two years

There may be any number of reasons why your child isn't sleeping well, but the commonest problems experienced by parents tend to have something to do with:

- a new baby joining the family;
- sibling rivalry – jealousy;
- juggling daytime sleeps;
- moving from cot to bed;
- children visiting their parents' bed in the night;
- travel and holidays;
- head-banging and rocking;
- children who are exceptionally early risers;
- inconsistency of parents' reaction to the problem.

Of course, in some cases a child's disturbed sleep pattern may also be as a result of never really having had any kind of bedtime routine established for her during the earlier part of her life. Once again, although this will inevitably be aided by better communication between you both, deciding on an appropriate bedtime routine and then putting it into practice will take some time and a fair amount of self-discipline on your part. (See Chapter 6 for more advice on bedtime routines.)

When a new baby joins the family

One of the most common times that families get into trouble with sleep routines is when a new baby arrives. It takes a brave parent to leave a baby to cry even for a few minutes at the risk of waking older children or, for that matter, to leave a toddler shouting for you just as the baby's got settled.

It is very easy for the focus of your activity to become nothing more than trying to hush whichever child happens to be waking up at the time. 'Soothe the toddler or she'll wake the baby' and 'Pick up the baby before she cries because we don't want to disturb the toddler' both become familiar phrases, repeated mantra-like over and over again! Instead of going to sleep, parents can end up spending almost the whole night vainly attempting to keep the house quiet.

Many families regularly play musical beds. By the time morning comes, parents have ended up in their children's beds, children are in their parents' bed and someone's usually given up all hope of sleep and has collapsed on the sofa. I know of one creative couple who, as a last resort, anticipated the arrival of 'night visitors' by having sleeping bags under their bed ready for the children to camp out in!

Other families have decided on Option 2 of the Top Seven (see Chapter 6) and just buy a big mattress and all jump in together. However, if you really don't want to share a bed with your children (even on an infrequent basis) you need to teach them to settle themselves without you. This, I'm afraid, will inevitably involve some noise in the short term. But if you're consistent and committed, Options 3, 4 and 5 of Chapter 6 shouldn't take more than a week to bring about some real changes. Often it is just a case of true grit and determination to make the option you've chosen work for you and your child.

'One child up in the night is bad enough,' I hear you say, 'but the thought of everyone awake is just too much!' But wait:

it may be horrendous for a few nights, but (and it's a very *big* 'but') those who have braved it say that it is well worth going through the pain barrier (and they include me). Short-term pain – long-term gain! And anyway, many children seem to be able to sleep through much louder noise than we anticipate – lots of parents are astonished when their older children don't wake up at all, despite the racket going on around them!

Only you appreciate how cheesed off you feel, but if you're really fed up, all I can say is do have a go. You might be pleasantly surprised, and if you stick to your plans sleep-filled nights may be just around the corner!

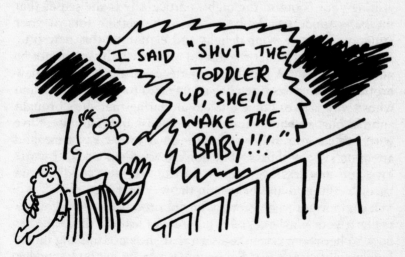

Top Tip: *Many parents are astonished when their older children aren't woken by the new baby – they can often sleep through much louder noise than we anticipate.*

Sibling rivalry

Soon after the arrival of a new baby, your toddler may start visiting your room in the night, particularly if she senses that the baby (understandably) seems to be getting lots of your attention. Despite your delight and elation at this new little person, to your toddler the arrival of a new baby might not be quite as thrilling! A toddler's experience on the birth of a new brother or sister has often been compared to that of a husband whose wife arrives home one day declaring that she's brought another husband home too. This new husband is going to 'live with us, eat our food and take up a lot of my time and attention', she enthuses. 'But don't worry,' she adds, 'I won't love you any less!' Suddenly we can see why toddlers can become confused and behave in the way that they do!

It's important to be gentle with your toddler, even if you are really at your wits' end. Give her a bit of leeway, then take her back to her room once she's seen that she's not missing much. Involving her is the key. For example, engage her by letting her help you look after the baby during the day, explaining that the baby needs a big sister's help. Star charts (see pages 143–4) may help keep her in bed at night-time, but ultimately she'll still want to check that she's not missing out on anything and that you still have lots of room in your heart for her.

 Top Tip: *Be gentle with your toddler and give her time to adjust to the presence of a new baby.*

Juggling daytime sleeps

As you will probably know from personal experience, even if you go back to sleep straight away, interrupted sleep is less satisfying than sleeping right through. It's no different for children; falling asleep for short periods in a buggy or the car is far less restorative than one long sleep lying down.

Now that she's older, it may be tempting to juggle with your child's daytime sleeps, but I would encourage you, as much as possible, still to try and allocate a regular time for them. Regular sleep can all too easily get sidelined if you are busy, or if there are other children's needs to attend to. But in actual fact, fixing a standard time for a morning or afternoon nap might be less hassle than you'd imagine; it's often just a matter of working out the best times to go for within the rest of the family's routine.

I've never been much of a juggler, but as soon as my daughter Ella started nursery, I took a crash course! She had to be there at 1 p.m., so my eighteen-month-old son Joe (who would be ready to go to sleep at midday for two hours), had to be persuaded to stay awake until after I dropped her off. Once home, Joe would have a couple of hours' sleep in his bed until it was time to pick Ella up again. On the bad days, however, he would fall asleep in his buggy on the way to nursery, sleep for twenty minutes or so, and then promptly wake up when he got home. He would then not be tired enough to get back to sleep in his cot but, having not had enough, would often be miserable and short-tempered. At 3 p.m. he would fall asleep again for another twenty minutes on the way to nursery, and this second twenty-minute 'power nap' (quite late in the day for him to sleep) would normally mean that I had to wave bye-bye to my precious evening.

Twenty-two-month-old Amy found it difficult to settle in her new cot bed. After several disturbed nights, Carol found that, as far as she could see, the only way to get her to sleep was to climb into the cot with her – literally! Carol slept one end, Amy the other. After several nights of this arrangement, Carol realised it was going to end up being a permanent solution unless she helped Amy to learn to fall asleep without her lying next to her.

She decided to follow the Checking option in Chapter 6. She made sure Amy had a new special 'grown-up girl's' cuddly blanket to hold, and explained that she wasn't getting into Amy's bed any more. Carol drew a rough sketch of herself and let Amy stick it next to her new cot where she could see it. When it came to bedtime, Carol would sing Amy a song, read her a story and then switch off the light and leave her room. Every five minutes Carol went in to Amy, who was crying steadily, and asked her to lie back down as it was time to sleep. The first evening, Amy fell asleep after eight visits from Carol and woke at 2 a.m. and 5 a.m. during the night. At 2 a.m. Carol went in every five minutes and Amy settled by 2.20. At 5 a.m., when Amy wasn't so tired, Carol visited again every five minutes and was kept up for forty minutes. The second and third nights were easier, with Amy only waking once in the night and falling asleep within two visits, and by the end of the week Amy was settling herself to sleep without any difficulty.

Moving from cot to bed

By the time she is two, you might want to start thinking about moving your child to a full-size single bed. When she does so, however, it's not uncommon for problems to arise as a result of her new-found freedom! There are a variety of methods you can employ to encourage her to stay put and stay safe in bed. The basic trick is to create a situation where there is more incentive to stay in bed than to get out. Additionally, if she knows that should she decide to keep climbing out (either to visit you while you're still up, or to come into your bed), you'll always return her to her bed, eventually she won't bother to leave.

 Top Tip: *Give her as much incentive as you can for her to stay in her own bed.*

Your child's bedroom (and your home) should already be as child-safe as possible, but once she has the freedom of being in a bed this is particularly important. For example, fix window locks, cover up unused electricity sockets, lock any medicines away and protect gas fires with a guard. Just about anything you can imagine her doing is good to guard against!

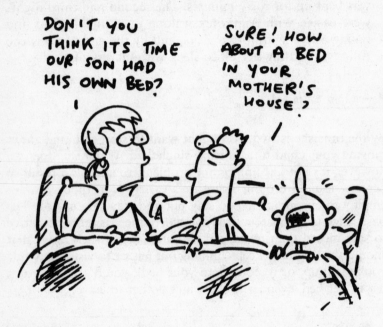

Who's been sleeping in my bed?

The new-found freedom of a bed gives your child more options for where she might sleep than ever before. Many parents wake up in the morning to find an extra little person in bed with them. Other parents wake up as their child joins them and search themselves for a less crowded place to spend the night, often doing a swap and opting for their child's empty bed!

Rajid (aged three) was waking several times a night, getting into his parents' bed. One night, while her husband was on night duty, Mum was woken by a noise and saw a ghost crossing her bedroom. On reaching the bed the ghost bent down on all fours and scurried under the bed. After a few minutes of silence, the ghost took off his bed-sheet disguise and carefully climbed into Dad's side of the bed, hoping not to be noticed. The ghost was returned to his room!

If your child's nightly appearances are getting you down and you really want her behaviour to change, the key thing, once again, is to be one hundred per cent dedicated to making it happen.

It's wise to think about the messages that you could be sending subconsciously to your child. If your bedroom door is open, with a well-lit hallway, your child might think you're inviting her in. You might want to try keeping the lights low for a few nights, and pulling your door nearly closed. And when you hear the patter of tiny feet don't delay in taking her straight back to her bed.

If you feel up to it, you could follow the example of some parents I know, who have got a chair and a duvet and told their child that they'll sit outside her room for a while. Others use a stair gate across the bedroom doorway so their child can't roam around at night. Both these options may work, but on the whole it's much better if you can help her to see that there's just no *point* in getting up, because nothing else ever happens other than being taken straight back to bed. When she eventually realises that there's absolutely nothing to be gained and that night-time really *is* for sleeping and that's it, she will soon lose her desire to leave her room.

One more thing: if your child does tend to be a night-time wanderer, it may be a good idea to put a stair gate across the stairs – children can easily become disoriented when they wake up, and you don't want any accidents.

Travel and holidays

Babies and children are more mobile than ever before. Most spend long periods of time in car seats, and many mums and dads can sing, word for word, every line of their particular version of the 'Sixty Minutes of Travelling Songs' tape which has taken up residence in the car's cassette machine!

The journey that can have a big impact on sleep patterns is the 'pick-up' car journey at the end of the day to school or carers. You look in the mirror to see if your youngest is OK and see, much to your alarm, that her eyelids are wearily drooping. You begin to mentally wave goodbye to your quiet 'evening to yourself' as you envisage hours of fruitless attempts to get her to go to bed later on. If you're lucky, you might be able to wake her before she's fast asleep, and if there's another adult in the car with you in order to help achieve this that's a great advantage. A hand-puppet, helpfully kept in the glove compartment ready to whip out at a moment's notice, is a useful tool for bringing instant alertness as she plays hide and seek. Another winner is the 'how long can my teddy bear balance on the passenger headrest?' game.

If you're on your own with a sleepy baby in the back seat, the only one I've got to work is 'Joe's not asleep, is he?' It's best suited to the over ones, and involves acting out that you believe your child is asleep. Teddy and a handful of imaginary passengers are told that he is asleep and are asked to be very quiet. If you start this before your child's nodded off he might stay awake for another ten minutes just wondering if you've completely lost your marbles!

Another suggestion: keep the back windows open (providing it's not raining), as he can't fall asleep so easily with the wind blowing through his hair. And finally, chocolate buttons also work for the truly desperate – if you haven't eaten them all first!

If you have to do a particularly long car journey, try to do it in the evening or at night-time if you can. Another tip is to try to get your child into his night-clothes before setting off, as this can make the transition to a bed at the other end much less disruptive. It's also good to bear in mind that journeys can often take longer than you anticipate and that children can dehydrate – so have a good supply of water on hand. Be prepared, too, for more stops on your journey than in the days before you had children.

Planes, trains and buses

The beauty of going by bus or train is that you'll often have so many people wanting to make your baby smile that the likelihood is you won't have the problem of her nodding off prematurely.

If you are taking a baby on an aeroplane, offer a bottle- or breast-feed as the plane takes off and descends, in order to release the air pressure in her ears. And don't be surprised if she's a bit cranky – babies can suffer jet lag and be just as miserable from travelling long hours as we can! If you're crossing time zones, remember to allow for time changes in her routines.

No more working for a week or two
Holidays with young children can provide precious memories for everyone – long, lazy days in the sun (hopefully!) with a chance to focus on the simpler things in life and recharge your batteries a bit. So the last thing you really want is for it to be stressful on the sleep front.

There seem to me to be two options. First, you can maintain as much of your normal home routine as possible, i.e. make tea at the usual time, give your child a bath before bed, etc. Or, second, you can create a new holiday routine that's more flexible, i.e. keeping your baby up later in the evening and letting her have a longer daytime sleep.

This second option works best if you are away more than a week – shorter holidays don't give you enough time to establish a new routine and make it worth the effort.

Don't forget to pack your child's usual comforts: dummy, teddy, toy Hoover (see page 95 if you don't believe me!), blanket, etc. If you are using an unfamiliar cot, make sure the mattress fits properly and that the frame is stable. Before bedtime, try to spend a good chunk of time with her in the room where she'll be sleeping – it'll help her to get accustomed to her surroundings.

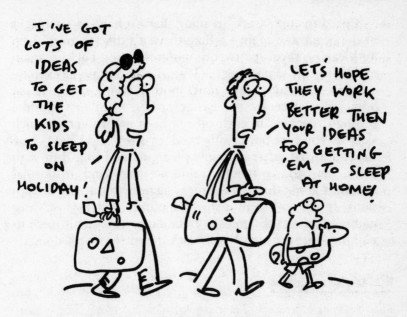

If you decide to opt for a new routine while on holiday, your child might be keen to continue with that routine when you're home. Alternatively, you may prefer to revert to the old ways of doing things as soon as possible.

Karin felt she knew what to do when her three boys woke in the night. She had used the Controlled Crying method with all of them at various times, and succeeded in establishing a bedtime routine which worked well for everyone. What she found tiring, though, was having to repeat the process whenever they got back from holiday, or if one of the children had been ill.

115

'I used to come back dreading that I'd have to start right at the beginning again – telling them it's time to go to sleep and leaving them for twenty minutes, going back in again and saying the same thing . . . It's just such a draining exercise – I can see why people don't bother trying and give in. Sometimes it seems the easier option is to just muddle through, sleeping in each other's beds just to get as much sleep as you can. But I really need my sleep and I soon came to realise that, after a couple of nights of being firm with them, the children would realise we were back to normal and start going through the night again without any disruptions. It can still seem a slog sometimes, but two or three nights of re-establishing the boundaries is a small price to pay for a proper night's sleep. It's definitely worth doing.'

Head-banging and rocking

Between five and ten per cent of children will bang or roll their heads in their cots before falling asleep during the first few years. It often begins as a comforting habit.

Rocking helps a child fall asleep. Sometimes the rocking can become quite violent, to the extent that the cot can shake and parents worry that their child might hurt herself.

Head-banging usually starts around the child's first birthday and often stops before her fourth. Reassuringly, there are no medical problems linked with it. It doesn't even indicate that your son or daughter may end up playing in a heavy rock band.

The key is to ignore the behaviour you want to prevent and praise the behaviour you want to encourage. Rocking or head-banging becomes a bigger problem when too much attention is given to it. Once your child realises he can attract more of your time and attention by keeping going, the behaviour will increase. In the same way as Sam's parents ignored her self-induced vomiting (see pages 96–7), once your child realises you're not taking any notice he's much more likely to stop naturally.

The dawn chorus - children who are early risers

This has to be one of the most frustrating sleep problems. What can you do when your child wakes at 5 or 6 a.m.? After all, it's still night-time really – surely this can't be called morning for at least another two hours!

There are two possible reasons why your child wakes early:

1 She has had enough sleep for her needs and is ready to face the day.
2 She hasn't had enough sleep yet, but has been woken up – by sunlight through the curtains, noise (the dawn chorus, traffic, the central heating switching on) or feeling cold.

If you think she's had enough sleep your options are:

- Swap a bit of your 'child-free' evenings for quieter mornings by making bedtime later.
- For the kind of child who will play on her own (and you won't know unless you try), have plenty of quiet toys and books available for her (perhaps a toy she hasn't played with for a while).

- Leave a drink and a biscuit within her reach, especially if she tends to be hungry when she wakes (although, admittedly, there is some risk that she may eat it at 2 a.m.).
- If she has yet to reach the stage where she can climb out, keep her in a cot (as opposed to a bed) for as long as possible. She is more likely to doze or play quietly if she can't get out of bed and go walkabout.
- Think about how tiring her day is – is she being ferried about in cars, sitting still a lot of the time? Is she getting a chance to get tired, not only physically but mentally too? Is this another reason to delay bedtime by half an hour or so?
- Your child's sleep needs are changing, so if you haven't done so already it may be time to drop the daytime sleep.

Not surprisingly, parents often bring their early risers into bed with them. A precious few more hours' sleep can be gained as your child snuggles next to you.

Go through a checklist to see if there's something stopping her falling back to sleep. If she's been coming into your bed for several weeks or months, the original reason for her doing so may well have disappeared and it's now just descended into being a habit. Treat this as you would if she was waking at 2 a.m. Decide on a way of managing her behaviour and stick to it.

Sometimes we don't even try the obvious. Nick, an old school friend of mine, told me about his son's early mornings:

Freddie, my eighteen-month-old, kept waking up at 5.30 a.m., and I couldn't stand it. A friend suggested I went into his room and told him it wasn't morning yet and to go back to sleep. I was amazed that I hadn't even thought of it, but it sounded so simple – surely it wouldn't work, would it? The next morning I tried it. Freddie looked surprised at first, then lay down in his cot and went back to sleep for another couple of hours! Bliss!

Bring on the rabbit

If these suggestions don't make any impact on your early riser, you could try using some props. Quiet ones are best – ones that won't wake your child should she miraculously sleep in longer! At least one high street shop sells a rabbit-shaped clock which opens its eyes and pricks up its ears at a time you choose. All you need to do is let your child know she can come into your room once Rabbit has woken up.

Another variation is putting a timer on your child's bedroom light. For the first two mornings, set the timer at the time she is waking up and tell her that she can come into your room once the light comes on. From then on, every couple of days, gradually extend the time when your child is allowed to come in to you by ten minutes. If she achieves your target (even though it might still feel like the middle of the night to you), be sure to praise and welcome her. Your attention is the best reward for keeping to her side of the bargain and gives her an incentive to keep going. It's important, too, to be specific about what you want your child to do – can she play in her room or elsewhere in the home? Is she allowed to come into your room and play quietly? Once she is older, star charts can be used to provide added incentive (see Chapter 10).

Seasonal variations

Persuading your child that it's still night-time when the sun is bursting through the window is tricky. I can only think of two tips. One, thick curtains with blackout lining! Two, explaining that the sun is only shining in the night-time because of a special request made by the flowers at this time of year: you can make up your own shaggy dog story or give them a short lesson in astronomy!

Consistency

It's easy to lose confidence in dealing with sleep disruptions if nothing seems to work.

For some, lack of consistency might be the main reason why they're not succeeding. After a couple of nights of struggling with one method, you're tempted to give in and move on to another. You're much more likely to chop and change if you've lost confidence in your own ability to sort out your child's sleep patterns. It's also much harder to stick to one way of getting children to sleep if you have a sneaky suspicion that another approach might magically do the trick overnight. But here's the truth – it won't. Call me boring, but all the evidence points to the fact that sleep patterns only change when parents are consistent over days, weeks and months. So my message is: as hard as it is, keep going and be consistent.

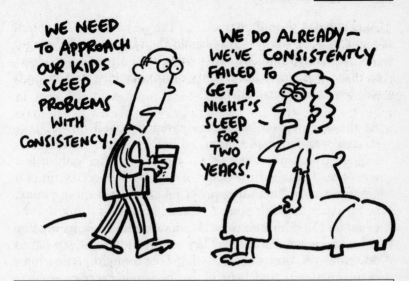

> ***Top Tip:*** *Whichever method you adopt to help your child learn to fall asleep, the key is to be one hundred per cent dedicated and one hundred per cent consistent.*

If you're looking for a powerful example of consistency in action, think about how you would react if you saw your toddler run across the road. Would you hesitate, wondering what to do? I doubt it. My guess is that you'd grab her without even thinking about it. However many times it happened (hopefully never), you'd react in exactly the same way. Total consistency and total confidence.

This is what should characterise the way that you respond at night to your baby – treat her in the same way night after night, and she will quickly learn what's expected of her. However, if she senses any uncertainty or anxiety in your approach it will have the reverse effect.

At the age of two, when his parents moved house, Jake started waking in the night asking for juice. At first this happened just once or twice a night, but after only a few weeks he'd reached the stage of waking five or six times a night, always demanding juice. Jake was still quite young, so his parents didn't want to leave him with a drink that he could just help himself to, and as a result their nights became more and more disrupted. They simply didn't know what to do. However, they did know that Jake thought getting juice in the night was so delightful that he would carry on waking unless they somehow changed the pattern.

They talked through the situation with their health visitor and agreed that they should sort it out as quickly as possible, rather than adopting the Softly Softly approach. They decided to let Jake choose a new cup for a night-time drink and then explained that, if he was thirsty in the night, he could have water in his special new cup. Jake's mum and dad felt their confidence rise even before the first night, because they said they could tell Jake had noticed their change in attitude. He could tell something was up.

Rather than diluting the juice or giving him less of it whenever he woke up, Jake's parents stopped offering juice altogether from the first night. Jake's initial reaction was to get cross. He would take the cup of water which was offered instead and throw it on the floor from his cot. Mum or Dad took each night in turn, said 'night-night' and walked out of Jake's room. They went back to him after he cried for twenty minutes and repeated the process. He fell back to sleep, usually after about forty minutes. By the third night Jake realised that the juice was not coming back (at least during the night), and by the fourth night he was getting himself back to sleep without either Mum or Dad's involvement.

Night-time fears

Some toddlers begin to have nightmares or night-time fears at this young age. Your child might be waking up – afraid of something they've seen or thought about – sitting up, looking terrified.

When Adam was two and a half he started waking up two or three times a night and would be crying and inconsolable for an hour. There didn't seem to be anything that triggered it. It started before we moved house but seemed worse afterwards. It was exhausting – the only way we could deal with it, because he cried so much, was to stay with him. Sometimes we wondered why we bothered, because he really would be inconsolable. We'd try really hard to wake him up and calm him down, but I think he was really only semi-conscious. We'd take him to the loo, which would sometimes wake him up enough to put him back into bed. By now, though, he'd often be alert enough to want one of us to stay with him until he got back to sleep, because he was frightened of being on his own. We stayed by his bedside while he fell asleep and would then go back to our own bed. The problem eventually resolved on its own after a few months, but it was very hard at the time.

These problems can be tricky to deal with, as your child's speech is unlikely to be developed enough for her to articulate exactly why she's so upset. Are there any other changes happening within your family that might be adding to your child's anxiety (i.e. moving house, tensions at home, etc.)? Can you give her more reassurance while those changes occur? Either way she'll need your comfort, and in some cases that's the best you can offer. Treat your child with extra care and kindness – as if she's younger than she is. Chapter 9 (see page 139) deals with nightmares in more depth.

When you've really had enough

In the middle of the night, when every part of you is longing to fall asleep, there is a fine line between loving and hating your child! Parents feel resentment and anger towards the child who is depriving them of sleep; but at the same time they also feel guilty for feeling like that. There are two things to try which may help to counteract these feelings. One is to watch your child sleeping (providing you've finally managed to get her to sleep) and the other is to write down one thing that you like about her – what she does that makes you smile. Both will help you to recapture your appreciation of your child – something that can quickly go out of the window when nights are bad.

It is at the times when you are on the edge, when you've given all you can give, that you realise that all parents have the potential to harm their children. Parents don't come pre-packaged marked as either 'good' or 'bad', with the bad ones appearing in the news for hitting their children while the good ones never put a foot wrong. We are all trying to do the best job we can. Often you'll be brilliant, but not always. And especially not when you're tired and feeling the pace. You'll shout louder, get angry at the least provocation, and you'll feel like a failure because you're letting yourself as well as your child down. But go easy on yourself – there's no mystery as to why you feel like this: if you haven't slept, you can't expect to be on top form.

If this rings lots of bells for you, try to find someone you can confide in. You're probably shocked that you feel so horrible towards your children, but there are professional people who won't be shocked at all, so get in contact with one of them – your GP, health visitor, Parents Anonymous, Parentline Plus or the NSPCC (telephone numbers at the back of the book).

 Top Tip: *If you are finding things really tough, don't wait to seek professional advice.*

The ball's in your court

Toddlers are great company, but they are on a very steep learning curve and are being asked to achieve an incredible amount in a relatively short period of time. They learn to walk (normally into puddles), climb (up your curtains), pull (things off your dressing table) and, best of all, they start to talk.

So changing sleep patterns at this age is a different, but winnable, ball game. Your child will be much more strong-willed and persuasive than previously, so decide what (if anything) you want to change, let your child know what's going to happen and then, most important of all, stick with it.

Special Situations

There are a number of situations where sleep problems are more common. This chapter offers some ideas on the following special circumstances:

- Children with disabilities or chronic illnesses
- Childhood illnesses
- Children with asthma
- Children with eczema
- Living in crowded accommodation
- Twins and multiple births
- Children with autism
- Children with Down's Syndrome
- Very active children
- Stepfamilies and looking after other people's children
- Nightmares, night terrors and sleep-walking

Children with disabilities or chronic illnesses

If your child has a disability or long-term health problem, he will require a lot of extra attention and time from you. The ideas in this book about creating clear boundaries, encouraging good sleep habits and instilling bedtime rituals are therefore even more pertinent for you and your child. When children are unwell or suffering in some way, parents naturally feel great worry and concern. As a result, it's much more difficult to be firm with a child. Consequently, children can learn some very bad habits. In order to avoid this trap, try and step back from your situation by writing a sleep diary – ask a friend or your health visitor to look through it with you with a fresh pair of eyes. It might be worth asking yourself if there is anything that you are trying to avoid in not dealing with your child's sleep problem. Maybe you can't stand listening to his crying or you don't feel ready to let him sleep in his own bed yet. Are there any medical reasons why your child's sleep problem can't be tackled? If you are in any doubt, ask your doctor's opinion. If he or she gives you the green light, take a good dose of courage and decide which of the seven top options suit your child and your family best (see Chapter 6). If you are at all worried about leaving your child to sleep on his own, I would recommend the Elastic Band option, as it is a method that is extra kind to both you and your child.

 Top Tip: *Don't be hesitant to tackle sleep problems if your child has a chronic illness or disability – you might be suffering bad nights unnecessarily. Are there any habits you can change?*

Childhood illnesses

Just like bats and hedgehogs, snuffly noses, post-immunisation temperatures and ear infections all seem to come out at night. And what's more, they often seem much worse during the small hours than during the day – possibly because you know there's not so much help easily accessible, or because you know you're likely to be up for some time getting your child comfortable.

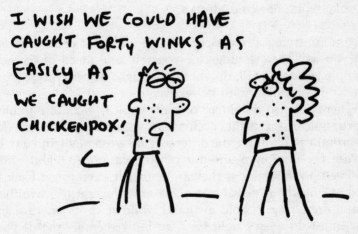

I WISH WE COULD HAVE CAUGHT FORTY WINKS AS EASILY AS WE CAUGHT CHICKENPOX!

Here are some things that can make a difference:

- Keep your child cool – but remove layers gradually, to prevent your baby becoming too cold.
- If your child is snuffly, put a couple of books under the feet of the cot, at the head end, so his head is slightly higher than his feet – he will find it easier to breathe.

- Did your granny ever make you lean over a bowl of boiling water with a towel round your head? Steam helps to clear the airways in the nose and throat, so either let your child into the bathroom when the shower is on, or repeatedly boil a kettle in the room where he sleeps, before you put him to bed. But avoid scalding: be quite sure your child can't get too close to the kettle or the steamy hot water.
- Offer lots of fluids (water, or breast or formula milk) as babies and children get thirsty quickly. Snuffly babies often like tepid, not cold, drinks.

If you are trying a new sleep routine and your child becomes ill, you will have to judge for yourself how much of the new routine you stay with, or whether it might be better to just put everything on hold until he recovers.

There are also a number of steps you can take to minimise disruption in the night, even when your child is unwell. It's important to reinforce the difference between night and day by giving the minimum amount of stimulation at night. Some people find this easy, as they are naturally keen to get back to bed as quickly as possible. Others are reluctant to leave their child, preferring to hold his hand while he drifts off to sleep. You must do what's right for you, but remember that if your child gets used to you holding his hand to fall asleep when he is unwell, he may be reluctant to stop when he's better. It can be difficult to decide when your child is well enough to get back into a routine after a period of illness – but once he is well, reintroduce your good sleep habits quickly in order to avoid slipping back into the old bad habits that you've worked so hard to break!

Children with asthma

Children with asthma tend to experience fragmented sleep – especially if their symptoms are poorly controlled. They are likely to wake with episodes of coughing, wheezing and breathlessness in the night. Many parents feel justifiably anxious that leaving their child to cry for any length of time may trigger an attack, and it is true to say that anxiety (yours and his) can make asthma symptoms worse. It is important that a child's asthma is controlled with adequate medication and that he is 'stable' before you begin to think about changing his night-time routine. The Softly Softly, All In Bed Together or Elastic Band options described in Chapter 6 are probably the ones which are best suited to encouraging your asthmatic child to sleep. The National Asthma Campaign is a good source of support and information; see their details at the back of the book.

Children with eczema

Children with eczema often have real difficulties at night. They find it especially difficult to settle once they wake in the night with hot, itchy skin. They can even end up making themselves bleed by scratching their skin without realising it. So if your child suffers from eczema, here are some key tips to remember:

- Use cotton bedlinen and nightwear – avoid man-made fibres.
- Don't let him get too hot at night – it'll make him more

131

itchy. Make sure his cot or bed isn't against a radiator.

- Use non-biological washing powder (there are conflicting views about using conditioner but, as my mother always says, 'if in doubt, leave it out').

- Use aqueous cream every four hours during the day when you can. Moisturisers absorb better on damp skin, so before bedtime let him have a short splash in the bath (avoiding bubble bath) before slapping on so much that you might even worry that he'll slip out of the bed at night! There's no point in attempting any of the seven options in Chapter 6 unless you've treated his skin first. Once his skin is more comfortable he will be more likely to sleep well. If aqueous cream doesn't seem to help and his sleep is being badly affected, your GP can advise more specific treatment and may refer you to a paediatric community nurse.

Your concern might also push you to check your baby more frequently than you really need to. This in itself may disturb him. It's a really difficult balance to get right, so don't be too paranoid about how you are doing. Most importantly, ask for some support with the nights, and take it in turns so you get some nights off.

There's no doubt that the parents of eczema sufferers know who their real friends are!

And there's also no getting away from the fact that, until your child's skin improves, eczema will seriously damage your nights. The Eczema Society offers excellent support and practical advice, and their details can be found at the back of the book.

Living in crowded accommodation

For parents living in one room, sleep routines can be very hard to impose. As children can't help but see and hear what happens after 'bedtime', it is very common for them to stay awake until their parents go to bed, late in the evening.

If your accommodation is cramped, you may use your child's cot during the day as a safe place for him to play. But as a result, he may then find it hard to associate his cot with going to sleep. Make the difference between night and day as obvious as possible. Use subdued lighting in the evening, have a regular bedtime routine and keep noise levels low.

Psychological boundaries are just as important and include:

- your body language – after bedtime, try not to look directly at him and also avoid sudden movements in the room;
- keeping your voice low or even whispering, until he's asleep. I know it's anti-social but, if you can, avoid conversation almost completely during this time. Don't have the TV on while he's falling asleep, even if you have the volume down – he'll want to watch it with you.
- being firm about bedtime routines. This can be very hard in cramped surroundings, and the temptation is definitely to let things slip because it's so difficult. But if you persevere, you'll be amazed at the results and you'll enjoy the fruits of your labour for years to come!

If you are in temporary accommodation and know that you are going to be rehoused soon, delay making any changes until you have moved – once you're settled you can really go for it!

Twins and multiple births

Twins, triplets or quads often have difficulty settling, for a variety of reasons. Sheer numbers mean that every aspect of childcare is more time-consuming, and bedtime is no different.

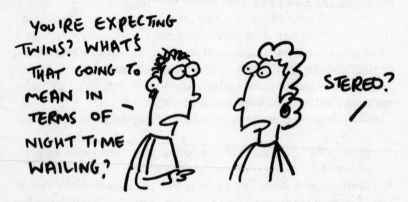

Many twins share the same cot. In fact, research shows that they are more likely to settle well if they are in close contact because it mimics the womb. The downside is that, in the first few months, the chances of the babies disturbing each other are fairly high. However, in time they will become accustomed to each other's cries and sleep through any disturbances. Having said that, some parents choose to separate their babies, so if your babies are waking each other regularly and you have the space don't feel pressured into keeping them together.

Twins or triplets can be settled for daytime and night-time sleeps either by putting them down to sleep at the same time or by dealing with each baby separately. On the whole, though, parents tend to find that if they establish a routine in which the babies feed and sleep together, it's easier for them to:

- have some time to themselves;
- hand the babies' care over to other willing volunteers;
- break the routine and be more flexible when the need arises.

If creating a routine doesn't sit easily with you and you'd prefer to discover your babies' natural rhythms instead, offer feeds on demand and let them sleep when they want. Inevitably there will be times when, as one baby goes to sleep, the other wakes up, so it's probably best only to try this approach if you have a good network of regular help and support available from family and friends who can help you grab a bit of time to yourself.

If you want to alter twins' sleep routines, all seven options described in Chapter 6 work for more than one baby!

Talk to parents who've been in the same situation. Shared experiences are often the most helpful. Contact TAMBA (Twins and Multiple Birth Association) for local contacts – their details can be found at the back of the book.

Children with autism

Autism is usually diagnosed during the pre-school years, and unfortunately sleep disorders are a common symptom. This can be due to many factors, including an autistic child's sensitivity to sound and general inability to relax. However, it is widely believed that, unlike with other children, attention-seeking is probably not a factor.

A sleep diary can be incredibly helpful in helping you to discover two important factors: first, the sleep problems you need to change, and second, which areas of your child's sleep disruption you can minimise.

Although they may take longer than the Checking or Controlled Crying options, the Softly Softly and Elastic Band methods are more suited to a child with autism. They are more likely to succeed in allaying any anxieties the child might have and are gentler on everyone involved. The National Autistic Society produces an excellent leaflet, entitled *Helping Your Child with Autism to Sleep Better*, in which it tells the following story:

> One child was unable to make the switch from sleeping in his parents' bedroom to sleeping in his own room. To deal with this, his parents slept in his room with him for a few nights and then moved to sleeping in the passage outside his room and slowly moved back to sleeping in their own bedroom. Although this approach may seem quite intrusive it worked because it acknowledged that the child's fears about sleeping alone were very real. Rather than forcing a confrontation it gave him the reassurance that his parents were never far away should he need them.

If you're not in contact with them already, the National Autistic Society offer specialised help, advice and support. If you'd like to speak to other parents of children with autism who've found creative solutions to sleep problems, a parent-run help-line service is also available, called Parent to Parent. See the contact list at the back for details of both organisations.

Children with Down's Syndrome

Children with Down's Syndrome tend to experience the usual sleeping problems of settling at bedtime and waking in the night. However, these children are also particularly prone to Obstructive Sleep Apnoea Syndrome (OSAS). The syndrome means that a child's sleep is frequently disrupted when the upper airway becomes blocked, preventing him from breathing. He then (unsurprisingly) wakes up, needing to breathe. This can happen hundreds of times each night, resulting in restlessness, loud snoring, coughing and choking noises. The cause of the problem should be investigated by an ear, nose and throat specialist, who may recommend treatment. This may well involve the removal of tonsils and adenoids.

The general advice and seven options for helping your child sleep better (listed in Chapter 6) are all suitable for a child with Down's Syndrome, but if he suffers from OSAS it is best to wait for the ear, nose and throat doctor's advice before following the Controlled Crying method. With an older child, rewarding good behaviour with your praise, attention and a motivator like a star chart (see pages 143–4) will bring better results than punishment.

Very active children

If you've got a child with a long-term sleep problem, the likelihood is that they are extremely exhausting, bouncy, Tigger-like characters. Active children tend to sleep less than placid types, and are more commonly boys.

A child who is diagnosed as either being hyperactive or

having Attention Deficit and Hyperactivity Disorder (ADHD) finds it especially hard to wind down enough to fall asleep easily. These children particularly benefit from firm boundaries that stay absolutely consistent night after night after night after night after night after night . . . For parents who find imposing discipline hard, having a child who needs strict guidelines can sometimes result in clashes. The key points to remember when this happens are:

- Try to keep calm yourself (sometimes this is the hardest bit). Speak to him in a firm voice with kindness in your eyes.
- Keep the home as calm as possible for a whole hour before bedtime, i.e. no loud music or TV, lower the tone of your voice (whispering can have an amazing effect on quietening the atmosphere), etc.
- Stick determinedly to the rules you've set.
- Ask for help – your GP or health visitor can refer you to more specialist support.

Stepfamilies and looking after other people's children

Persuading reluctant children to sleep is difficult for most parents, but it can be especially hard if you are not the child's natural parent. It's difficult to impose your discipline on another person's child. If you are a parent within a newly combined family, talk with your partner about how and where you expect the children to sleep – his or her expectations regarding bedtime routines might be very different from your own. The important thing, as in every family, is to decide together as a couple and maintain a united front. If one of you says something different or you don't back each other up, you are asking for trouble. Agree on a plan and then stick to it.

When new families are formed, there are adjustments for the children as well as the adults involved. There may be house moves, new step-parents and new children to get to know and build trust with, as well as new routines or new schools. It's important to maintain as much of your children's or step-children's habits and routines as possible, and that includes bedtime boundaries. If there are older children in your new family, try to involve them in agreeing on basic rules. Step-children coming to stay can cope with different sleep routines in different homes – they can adapt to yours when visiting your home, as long as you agree on what the basic rules are. Lots of listening, talking and being honest and patient can help, too. Parentline Plus offer a parent telephone service if you'd find it helpful to get more support in this area. Their details are at the end of the book.

Nightmares

Nightmares are common, and most children experience them at some stage. They:

- occur in the Rapid Eye Movement light stage of sleep (see page 44), during the last two-thirds of the night;
- are more common in families who have a history of nightmares;
- are unlikely to be linked with any emotional problems;

- usually sort themselves out and stop on their own;
- can sometimes be triggered by what a child has seen on television, in a book, etc.

At the age of five, Hayley watched *Snow White and the Seven Dwarfs* at school. She didn't like the evil witch and, as a result, had nightmares. Even just seeing a film clip of the dwarfs would trigger off the association with the witch, and the nightmare would return. Her parents didn't let her watch or read the story of Snow White for several years – even the parts of the film that were not frightening, simply because any pictures of the film would trigger the nightmares.

Often children wake up screaming, repeating phrases like 'go away', 'no', 'no more', etc., as if they are recalling something that has happened before. You can try to wake your child up gently to reassure him as much as possible. If he can remember the dream he may be reluctant to go back to sleep without your comfort. He may want to explain what it is about – let him talk but *don't* ask lots of questions that might make things worse! You may like to give him suggestions as to what to do if they recur (e.g. tell the monster your daddy is going to chase him away if he's nasty).

Your main job is to reassure him that although his fears *seem* real his dreams are not, and you can help him learn the difference. Your confidence in his ability to cope with the nightmares will help him enormously. Try to keep tabs on what your child is watching on TV, reading, or seeing on his computer – avoid things that will compound his fears. I have to confess that I am still scared by the child-catcher in *Chitty Chitty Bang Bang*!

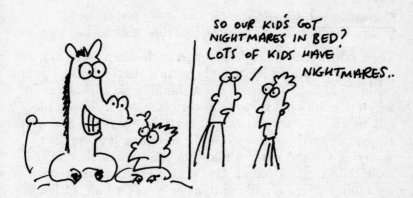

Night terrors

Despite this being a very frightening experience to witness, a child who suffers from a night terror is not aware of it happening and will not remember it in the morning.

Night terrors are caused when the emotional centre of the brain stays active while the rest of the brain is in deep sleep. The child screams, appears terrified and is often confused and hard to wake. In fact, it is better if you don't try to wake him. Instead, go to him as quickly as you can and stay with him while his fear subsides. Night terrors:

- are rare, much less common than nightmares;
- occur in the first few hours, in deep sleep;
- can happen when a child is unwell or when there have been changes in his routine such as during school holidays, after trips or when starting a new school.

141

Sleep-walking and sleep-talking

These both occur in the deepest part of the sleep cycle, too, and in some ways are similar to night terrors. Sleep-walking is more common in boys and has a strong family link. It is not usually a sign of emotional stress or disturbance. Most sleep-walking/talking children are unaware of what they're doing and won't remember anything about it in the morning. It is usually m worrying for the parents than the child when they disco their child trotting round. One parent heard a disturbance in the middle of the night and thought it was a burglar. Finding her child standing in the kitchen holding a tea towel was a shock in more ways than one!

Sleep-walking is caused by the movement centre in the brain remaining active during sleep. Older children have even been reported trying to climb out of windows or open the front door, so ensure your child's safety by fixing window locks and stair gates. Most sleep-walkers eventually stop on their own, although there are many adults who still wander round the house at night wearing pyjamas and a glazed expression!

For anyone who finds themselves facing one of these 'special' situations – whatever it may be – the key thing to work towards is consistency and routine. If you are still getting very little sleep, don't be afraid to seek a bit of extra help – it's what the health professionals are there for. And remember, however special your situation is, don't let it prevent you from getting the sleep you need and the sleep you deserve.

Three to Five Years

Now for some good news! Changing children's sleeping routines becomes much easier the older they get! Their language and understanding is more developed and they are therefore more open to change. It's a good idea to give your child incentives to change her sleeping habits, by rewarding good behaviour with praise and attention. Talking of which . . .

Stickers and star charts

Star charts are an excellent method of motivating three- to five-year-olds to change their sleep habits. To make a star chart, take a piece of paper and write the seven days of the week down one side, making a space next to each day for a sticker. It's important that your child should feel it's *her* chart (rather than yours) so let her decorate it however she chooses – if she wants to glue pine cones and sweet wrappers round the edge, fine! Then she needs to choose a packet of stars or stickers – the more excited she is about them, the better.

Now that's done, ask yourself what it is that you're wanting her to do. It has to be clear for her to understand and achievable for her age. Each morning, if she's managed to do what you've asked, give her lots of praise and let her stick a star or sticker on the chart. The key is to praise and motivate her enough so that she wants a sticker every morning. Once she can see her success in front of her, it will act as a catalyst. On the days she doesn't manage it, just leave the space on the chart blank, but on no account ever make a fuss about the fact that she hasn't been successful. Children respond much better to rewards and praise than to punishment, so however hard you might find it, praise her good behaviour rather than highlighting the bad. Don't be tempted to put a cross on the days she hasn't succeeded, and equally, never remove any stickers from the chart once she's earned them.

If after three or four days she hasn't managed to earn any stickers, check that you're not expecting too much too soon and revise her goal. Say, for example, your child is waking three times a night and coming into your room – it is too much to expect her suddenly not to wake you at all. In this case, take smaller steps that are easier for her to achieve. Start by giving her a sticker if she wakes you twice a night. Once she's succeeded in doing that for four or five days then you can make it harder, by offering her a sticker when she wakes you only once. Make the first steps achievable so she can enjoy her rewards – then gradually raise the stakes when she's got into the swing of it.

If motivation begins to wane, you can offer extra treats as an added incentive. If your child manages to get three stickers in a row, for instance, let her do something she really enjoys, like playing in the park or going swimming. Children love their parents' attention, so often the best reward you can give is your time. Other ideas could be to choose what to eat for tea (even if it isn't what you fancy!) or to visit a friend. Rewards should be fun, but don't have to be big or expensive.

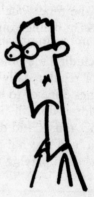

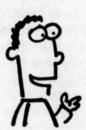

SURE I'D LIKE SOME 'SLEEP STICKERS' — I COULD STICK THEM OVER YOUR MOUTH SO YOU'D STOP GOING ON ABOUT SLEEP!

One word of warning: don't get carried away and offer rewards that are beyond a child's ability to focus on or earn. For instance, don't expect a three-year-old to be motivated enough to collect three weeks' worth of stickers before receiving a Barbie doll. She will need far more immediate rewards initially, and only as she grows older will she be able to understand the concept of building points to get a reward.

> **Top Tip:** Agree on realistic sleep 'targets' for your child and praise her whenever she manages to hit them. Incentives like star and sticker charts can also help.

What, no lunch break?

By the time your child reaches three she is likely to be pretty good at telling you exactly what she likes and dislikes. And that list of 'dislikes' will often include the daytime nap! Many parents (including me) miss this dreadfully, having become accustomed to a regular daily break from childcare in order to get a few things done or to have some time to themselves. However, some children do still benefit from an hour's rest after lunch, while other mums and dads try to keep the idea of the daytime ritual of a 'nap', even if all it actually means is that their child stays in her room playing with her dolls or daydreaming.

> **Top Tip:** We all need a bolt-hole to escape to for a bit of peace and quiet every now and then, so create a space in the day for your child to have a little time to herself.

Tiring her out

At this age, children need a fair amount of brain 'stretching', as well as physical activity, to tire them out. If you think your child might not be tired enough to sleep, combine running and jumping with getting her to work hard at thinking and imagining things. Ask her questions about a picture in a book or magazine, collect leaves and stones to make a mud castle in the park and pretend she is the queen in charge with you as her servant (you might feel you've been playing that role for some time already!).

 Top Tip: Don't forget, your child will need to be active during the day, both physically and mentally, to help her to be ready for a good night's sleep.

You'll probably notice that certain stages make your child much more tired than normal, such as when she starts to attend playgroup or nursery. This is because her brain and body are both being stretched more than ever before. And everyone knows that it's an exhausting business making playdough pirate ships and pretending to be Fizz from the Tweenies all morning!

But you were always such a good sleeper...

Some children may have slept like a log since day one only to start experiencing serious problems as they reach the pre-school stage. If this happens, it can be quite a surprise for the parents. But one study has shown that one in ten three- and four-year-olds were still waking frequently, so you are not alone!

A sudden change to disturbed nights in three- to five-year-olds can be due to any one of a number of common reasons.

Fear of being left

Children at this age can often feel anxious about something they've seen on TV, heard in a story or seen in a book. They are also sensitive to our moods – if you've had bad news (at work or in the family), your child will notice and it could affect her sleep. Children can feel responsible for your mood. Honesty is the best policy, and if you can give a simplified explanation rather than pretending that everything is normal it can help.

Your child may also learn to say that she is frightened, knowing that you're more likely to stay in her room, let her get into your bed or offer drinks or food. This has nothing to do with fear but is instead a great way of manipulating you. Whether there is something genuinely frightening her or whether she is just learning to manipulate what happens at night, the advice is the same:

- Acknowledge fears that are genuine and try to minimise them. 'I understand the shadow might look frightening. Shall I close the door a bit and see if it makes a difference?' or 'I didn't like that bit of the video either, it was scary. But it's not real, it's a story.'
- Try to avoid getting into the habit of 'shooing away' the ghosts from under the bed, because then you'll be confirming that there are ghosts under the beds to shoo away. Think about whether there may be any television programmes or computer games she is watching that might make the situation worse.
- Never dismiss or laugh at her fears. All this will do is ensure that she is less forthcoming about them in the future.

148

These are just examples – you need to find ways of reassuring your child that come naturally to you. At time of writing, my son is reluctant to fall asleep because he says that he is scared of the dark. I've found myself explaining that the birds have gone to sleep in their nests and Fudge, our next-door neighbour's dog, is asleep in his basket. This has led to twenty questions about the bedtime rituals of just about every animal he knows! By the time we've been through worms, rabbits, dogs, cats, snails, slugs, frogs and bugs, he's realised that if *they* are not scared of the dark and are already asleep, then maybe *he* should give it a go, too. It's working this week, at least!

If your child has had fears for quite a while then the Softly Softly, Elastic Band, Checking or All In Bed Together methods described in Chapter 6 should do the trick.

 Top Tip: *If your child is afraid of being left, never dismiss or laugh at her fears. She needs you to reassure her.*

An open invitation to your bed

If you want to encourage your child to stay in her room, a brightly lit corridor and Mum and Dad's wide-open bedroom door send completely the wrong message. You may as well put up a sign saying 'Children who want to climb into bed with us, this way please'! Use low wattage bulb nightlights in the corridors and pull your bedroom door nearly shut if you don't want to encourage visitors in the night. If you're sharing the bedroom with your child, small nightlights that plug into a socket might reassure her.

How you react to your child's behaviour will communicate your limits and what you expect. Try to keep your reaction to a minimum. If you repeatedly return your child to the same place to sleep, she'll eventually realise you mean it and will be more likely to settle without you.

 Top Tip: *Think about the unspoken messages that you may be sending to your child... She may think that, although you say, 'Stay in your bed!' you're really inviting her into yours.*

Refusing to go to bed

You can't *force* a child to sleep any more than you can get her to eat a bowl of slug stew! You can, however, ask her to stay quietly in her bedroom. But you should give her plenty of warning that bedtime is coming up – and not be unfair enough to expect her to drop everything the minute you say 'bed'.

Wherever your child sleeps, whether in a room shared with you or other children or on her own, let her feel she owns some of the space around the bed. Let her 'decorate' this space with pictures or personal things that are important to her. If you're feeling brave, let her get involved in painting the room where she sleeps! She's more likely to want to go to bed if she has a vested interest in it. Star charts (see pages 143–4) may also help to get through a particularly sticky patch of stubbornness.

> **Top Tip:** *Let her make the space around her bed a nice place to be – in her opinion, at least!*

Children need to get to a point where they believe that being in bed has got to be fun, so do most of the 'nice' bedtime routines once your child is actually in bed – reading, singing, telling each other jokes, etc. It can become a very special time when she can enjoy your full attention, even for ten minutes, to talk about her day or what's on her mind as she relaxes. If she particularly enjoys this time with you, why not make bedtime half an hour earlier, so you're not rushed?

And talking of making bedtime earlier, here's a common complaint from parents of pre-schoolers . . .

Bedtime is getting later and later

If you let bedtime drift later and later, your child will get the message that this is OK. If you're fed up with not having any evening left for yourself and want bedtime to be earlier, try and reintroduce it gradually. Make bedtime ten minutes earlier than normal for a few nights, then another ten minutes earlier and so on until bedtime is when you want it to be.

Tracey, who was four years old, refused to go to bed until she heard Big Ben chime at the beginning of *News at Ten*. Her parents were beside themselves because they knew she was getting really tired. They found a creative solution by videoing the news and then playing it earlier and earlier until she was going to sleep at 7 p.m. Tracey was none the wiser but much better behaved and happier as a result of getting the sleep she needed!

Becoming dry at night

Most children learn to 'hold on' during the night, or wake up and use the toilet, between the ages of three and five. However, one in every six five-year-olds is still not 'dry'. Dry nights rarely happen instantly, and children will occasionally have 'accidents' after having been dry for some time. An unexpected wet bed may be a sign that your child is worrying about something or is overtired. Be sensitive to any changes to your child's environment and be quick to reassure her.

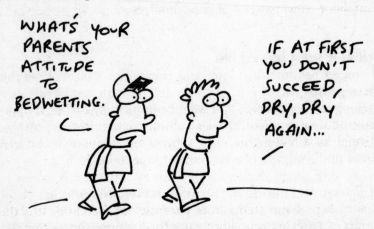

WHATS YOUR PARENTS ATTITUDE TO BEDWETTING.

IF AT FIRST YOU DON'T SUCCEED, DRY, DRY AGAIN...

Keep your night-time contact to the minimum. Keep a potty by her bed so she can nip out of bed, do a wee and then return to bed quickly. This way she won't wake up as much as with a full-blown trip to the loo, and she might not need to disturb you at all.

She might need help with learning to stay dry at night, but that doesn't mean she has to hold your hand for half the night while she goes back to sleep. As before, remain as dull and boring as you can – or you'll find yourself in deep early-morning negotiations that wouldn't seem out of place in a UN Security Council meeting! Try the Softly Softly approach descri-bed in Chapter 6 if she's finding it really difficult to get back to sleep or you're worried she'll wake other family members.

 Top Tip: *Use incentives and rewards for good behaviour, but give as little attention as possible to the behaviour you're trying to avoid.*

Illness and holidays

During illness or holidays away, children often enjoy their parents staying with them at bedtime while they fall asleep. Parents usually don't mind at bedtime, but when their children wake in the night and creep into Mum and Dad's bed they get cross with them, expecting them to be able to fall asleep in their own bed during the night. As we've seen in other chap-ters, this problem stems from parents, not the child. It is the result of applying one set of rules for bedtime and an entirely different set for night-time. As a result, children are sent, and therefore receive, mixed messages. It's no wonder that, if in doubt, they choose the most comfortable option – snuggling in with Mum or Dad!

When Warren was four he went on holiday, sharing a bedroom with his parents. He had been a good sleeper since birth. He came back from holiday having enjoyed sleeping with his parents and decided that it would be a good habit to stick with! Warren managed to keep this holiday habit going for four months, but by then his parents decided that they had had enough.

Warren's parents found it very difficult to leave him crying in his room, so they decided to take gradual steps towards him sleeping in his own room through the night again. They started by talking with him about going to sleep without Mummy or Daddy in his room, like he used to. They managed to get him to agree to settle in his bed while one of them sat by his bedroom door, explaining that they would stay there until he fell asleep. After four nights of this they showed him the chair just outside his room where his parents would sit while he fell asleep. If he got out of his bed they said they would shut his door. This gave him enough incentive to stay put in bed while still knowing they were nearby. After several nights they explained they would sit on one of the stairs and Warren could choose which step they would sit on. He used one of his favourite stickers to mark the step. They then explained that they would move down one step each night.

This very gradual process was hard work, but Warren's parents felt each step was achievable and, more importantly, it didn't involve Warren crying for long periods of time. Each night he stayed in bed and settled without help, Warren would receive a dinosaur sticker the following morning to put on a special chart that he'd drawn. This gave him an added incentive. Several times his parents had to take him back to his bed, telling him that it was night-time and to go to sleep, but their consistency paid off. Within three weeks Warren had settled back into his old pre-holiday routine.

Hospital visits and accidents

Unsurprisingly, some children find that their sleep is disrupted after an accident or having been in hospital. Let her talk about what has happened and make time to really listen. It may be upsetting to hear your child's feelings, but take her concerns seriously. If she knows you are listening, it will be the first step in calming her fears. If you need further support and advice, ask your GP or health visitor.

Treats and occasional nights breaking the rules

It's an unglamorous job being the one who lays down the rules when trying to get sleep patterns sorted, so, to lighten things up, remember that rules are made for breaking (if only occasionally) and change the routine for a night. Let your child stay up late as a treat and have a midnight feast (at 10 p.m., if you put the clocks forward). Remember, though, that every child is different, and be aware of how flexible yours is. Some children cope better with changes in routine than others, so be sensitive to your own child's needs.

Earlier today I spoke on the phone to Diane, a friend of mine, and told her that I was writing a book. 'What's it about?' she enquired.

'Getting your child to bed,' I answered.

'If only that was my problem,' she sighed. 'I can't ever get mine *out* of bed!' Diane is the mother of a normal fourteen-year-old. So even if you are struggling, take heart – it won't last for ever. One day you'll wonder what the problem ever was!

 Top Tip: *You may be surprised when bedtime starts to get easier. Stick to your plan and you'll soon be saying, 'I wish I'd done it months ago!'*

Once at School

Still sleepless after all these years . . .

Some things never change! You couldn't persuade your new-born baby to sleep more than he needed to, and you've probably realised that you can't do much more to persuade your six-year-old, either! The amount of sleep children need tends to lessen by about fifteen minutes with each birthday. As a rough guide, a five-year-old will need eleven hours and a sixteen-year-old eight and a half – although you may find this hard to believe as you struggle to get your sleepy teenager out of bed to go to school.

If your child only needs eight hours' sleep, there's not much point in expecting him to sleep for any more! But you can still establish boundaries at bedtime. At the end of the day, many parents feel they need a little time to themselves and so set up a routine of sending their child to his room to get ready for bed, even though he's not ready to fall asleep. Each parent needs to decide for themselves where these boundaries lie – whether your child has to actually go to bed, or whether he can play in his room. However, remember that leaving your child to play with a brother or a sister is only advisable if you know that they will play quietly and will not end up requiring your services as a referee!

It's not uncommon for older children, suddenly, and inexplicably, to have trouble going to sleep. This can last for days and sometimes weeks, and the best (and only) remedy is to provide as much reassurance as you can in an attempt to allay any fears he may have.

> Sarah had no trouble sleeping until she was nine. Then one night she couldn't get to sleep and lay in bed listening to all the noises in the house. By midnight the whole family was asleep – except Sarah, who became quite fearful about being the only one left awake.
>
> The same thing happened the next night, and within a week a pattern had established whereby Sarah would lie in bed at night and become more and more panicky about not being able to sleep.
>
> Sarah's parents provided lots of reassurance as Sarah went through this difficult patch. There was no easy solution but eventually, several months later, Sarah came to terms with her own fears and started sleeping normally again.

'But I don't want to go to bed yet!'

No one wants to miss out, and you can hardly blame a child for not wanting to go to bed, especially if there's something good on the TV and everyone's laughing and having a good time downstairs. So turn the TV down and try to be a bit less raucous or you'll soon hear the patter of little feet and see a pair of bleary eyes peering round the door!

Try and ensure that your child's bedroom is an attractive place to be. That doesn't mean you have to turn it into Disney World, but it does mean that it needs to be somewhere he will want to snuggle down. And however tempted you may be from time to time, avoid using early bedtime as a punishment. Create a cooling off corner in another room and then put him to bed when you're back on good terms. Don't ever let your child see bedtime as a punishment.

Life's little incentives!

Sticker charts, especially with added end-of-week rewards, come into their own with children of infant school age. When your child manages to achieve what you've asked him (say, for instance, staying in his room quietly after 8 p.m. or, if he's an early riser, not disturbing anyone else until a specific time in the morning) he gets an immediate reward the next morning in the form of a sticker. Let him draw up a sticker chart and choose the type of sticker – even if it's a blood-sucking alien from outer space (at least it isn't going to be staring at *you* from the wall all night!). He can then build up points each day, so that when he's got seven stickers in a row he can have an extra reward, such as a magazine/comic or a trip to the chip shop. Probably without realising it, you are already doing something similar yourself, but instead of being given dinosaur stickers you get loyalty points from the local supermarket. Life is all about incentives!

Give one hundred per cent praise and attention in the morning and very little at night, and he'll soon realise when's the best time to come and see you!

Distraction can be quite useful:

One five-year-old who couldn't get to sleep one night came into the sitting room where his dad was watching television.
'Dad, I can't get to sleep.'
'OK. Well, I tell you what, if you go back to bed but stay awake all night I'll give you a pound in the morning.'
The boy quickly shot back to bed, and when his dad went to see him twenty minutes later he'd fallen fast asleep.

Children of all ages are quick to tune in to incentives:

When Anthony was ten and his brother Stuart was eight, Stuart became frightened in the night and asked his mum and dad if he could sleep in their room. They told him to go back to his own bed to sleep. He then asked Anthony if he could sleep on his floor, to which his brother agreed. Several months later, when Stuart had his birthday, he said to his mum that he was cross with Anthony. When asked why, Stuart explained that he thought Anthony shouldn't charge him today because it was his birthday. 'Charge? What charge?' his mum asked. Stuart had been paying Anthony 5p a night for the privilege of his company. (Not surprisingly, Anthony has grown up to be an accountant!)

Bedwetting

Bedwetting at night is not unusual in children up to seven years old. In fact, five per cent of eight-year-olds still wet the bed three or more times a week. This can be for all sorts of reasons:

- *Family history* – if the parents weren't dry at night until the age of six or seven, their children are unlikely to be, either.
- *Development* – your child's control of his bladder hasn't developed fully yet.
- *The age of your child* – if you are comparing your child's development with that of his classmates, you should take into account where your child was born within the school year. A five-year-old born in September will understandably be ahead of a five-year-old born the following June.
- *Regression* – approximately half of five-year-olds who are bedwetting have been dry in the past but have slipped back. It is good to ask yourself why this might be happening.
- *Emotional factors* – bedwetting can be linked with a child's emotional problems, such as moving house or the break-up of the family.

Encourage your child to take responsibility for recognising when his bladder is full, and for reaching the toilet in time. Once he's mastered these good toilet habits during the day, the nights will often follow suit.

Try taking your child to the toilet before bedtime and again before you go to bed. Make minimal fuss over changing sheets, and certainly don't be distracted from getting back to your bed as quickly as possible.

Praise him in the morning for any dry beds, but never criticise him for an accident. Getting frustrated or angry at wet nights will only make your child anxious, and consequently makes the situation worse.

Top Tip: *Give plenty of praise when he gets it right, but never criticise him for bedwetting 'accidents'.*

There's a lot of emotional angst created over wet beds – especially for the person who ends up washing the sheets! But remember, as traumatic as it is for you, it's twice as upsetting for your child, so be gentle.

Sleepovers

Whoever coined the word 'sleepover' was clearly deranged! Sleepovers have very little to do with sleep but are very popular once your child reaches a certain age. Sleepovers are basically an excuse to get together with friends, giggle the night away and then enjoy breakfast together. This pastime is even more popular with girls than boys, so if you have sons sit back and for every weekend you don't have a sleepover count your blessings – or the number of extra hours' sleep you'll gain over those of us with daughters!

Top Tip: *Sleepovers are great fun, but when planning when they're going to happen, remember that they normally involve very little sleeping!*

Below are a few tips which might help make those sleepovers a little less chaotic.

Sleepovers at home

The more children you invite to stay for the night, the less sleep the whole house will get! Don't invite more children than you can manage.

- Don't have a sleepover if you know you will be very busy the following day.
- Speak to all the parents of the visiting children and find out what to do with their children in case they don't settle/have nightmares/unexpected temperatures/asthma attacks, etc. This is especially important if you don't know the children very well. Forewarned is definitely forearmed.
- Be flexible. Sleepovers are meant to be fun, and your child will not want to go to sleep too early. However, it's quite reasonable to set a time by which you want the 'happy campers' to settle down. Going into the bedroom and calmly turning off the lights at a given hour helps reinforce this point.
- Midnight feasts are great fun, but they don't have to happen at midnight!

Sleepovers away from home

- If your child has been invited to a sleepover but is reluctant to go, don't force him. Some six-year-olds will happily swan off with their sleeping-bag, while others don't want to sleep away from home until they're ten.

- If your child is uneasy about staying with a particular family, listen to what he says and keep him at home.
- Always give your child an opt-out. Tell him that you will pick him up – whatever time it is – if he really can't settle and wants to come home.
- Let the host parent know all your child's particular needs – see above.
- Go home and have a night off (hopefully!).

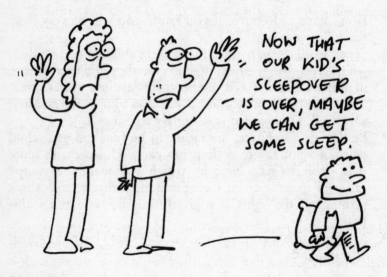

NOW THAT OUR KID'S SLEEPOVER IS OVER, MAYBE WE CAN GET SOME SLEEP.

Exam nerves

I recently asked a fourteen-year-old what she thought she needed most at exam time; the answer was for her parents to 'cut her some slack'. I thought she might have said she needed a good ten hours of undisturbed sleep – but no. Exams begin in primary school and they go on for ever, it seems. Anxiety, especially in older children, can cause difficulty in sleeping as well as disturbed nights – you can probably remember a few yourself!

As a parent, your role is to encourage and support at exam time, and therefore to help your child keep the whole exam procedure in perspective. Be relaxed, even if your own stomach is churning in sympathy, and encourage your child to stick to his bedtime routine. Nagging your child the night before he sits his exam is not a good idea – if he hasn't done his revision, it's too late, and in any case what he really needs most is a good night's sleep, not an ear-bashing!

> **Top Tip:** Exams can bring pressure for everyone. As a parent, it's your responsibility to encourage and support your child, and to encourage him to stick to his bedtime routine.

Sleepovers and parties are not advisable just before exam time. One parent allowed her daughter to go to a sleepover two nights before SATs and was horrified to discover that she hadn't gone to sleep until 4 a.m. The parent really only had herself to blame. The parties can wait until after the exams – they'll almost certainly be much more fun when the kids can really let their hair down!

Two final suggestions. If your child is a bit more tense and bad-tempered than usual, heed the advice of that fourteen-year-old and make some allowances. Do all you can not to add to your child's pressure. And second, recognise that it's normal for parents to get exam nerves, too. However, it's your job to work hard not to pass your anxieties on to your child, especially near bedtime.

Over-stimulation

We all know what it's like to watch a late-night thriller on the telly and then find that we can't sleep. Exactly the same applies for children. If, as bedtime approaches, your child watches an action-packed TV programme or battles aliens on the computer, don't be surprised if it takes him a while to settle down for the night. Researchers have found that watching television before bedtime results in children going to sleep later and for a shorter time. So think twice, or maybe three times, about that idea of allowing them to have a TV in their bedroom. In my opinion there are at least a hundred reasons why it's not a great idea.

 Top Tip: None of us finds it easy to get to sleep if our mind is buzzing – one of many reasons why a TV in your child's bedroom may not be such a great idea.

The 'just five more minutes' ploy is a popular and effective delaying tactic. Every child knows that five minutes can easily turn into fifteen or twenty or even half an hour. No child will willingly stop an enjoyable experience, especially if there is little or no structure which says 'bedtime'. So it's important to keep plugging away at a routine so your child knows what time he's expected to go to bed. But do be flexible as your child grows. If he continually complains that he's going to sleep far earlier than his friends (and he surely will!), have a chat with the other parents and find out what time his friends really do go to bed. You may be surprised!

As your child gets older, the responsibility for bedtime should shift, on a sliding scale, from you to him. Your long-term aim is obviously to encourage him to set the boundaries for himself as he slowly becomes more independent. You may think you'll never get there, but you will. And you'll know you've hit the jackpot when one day he puts himself to bed, not because you've told him to but simply because he's tired and wants an early night!

On Your Marks, Get Set . . .

Are you ready to take the plunge? If you're feeling revved up to create big changes in your family's sleep habits, it's likely your child will have already noticed a difference in your attitude. She'll be aware there's change in the air! You're already halfway there, so whatever you do, don't stop now!

On the other hand, if you've reached this chapter feeling faint-hearted and wondering if you're up to the task, here are some ways to build up your confidence and increase your chances of success.

Blame it on the weather man . . .

It's not unusual for parents to blame themselves if their children have sleep problems. However, as we've seen, all babies and children have periods of being restless at night for different reasons. This book isn't aiming to make you worry about the past: it's simply designed to help you help your child to learn good sleep habits, so that those periods don't last any longer than they need to. Don't waste time and energy thinking about what you might or might not have done wrong – look to the future and to the joy of sleeping all night long!

It's good to talk

It's really important that you find people to give you support during a time when you are trying to change your child's sleep habits. Friends, family, your health visitor or other parents who've got the 'been there, done that' T-shirt can all offer invaluable support, so get them on your side. Having someone to listen to you talk about your situation can help you identify more clearly what needs to be tackled and how to go about it consistently each night. Think of it as the sleep equivalent of a personal fitness trainer – celebrities have personal fitness trainers to motivate them, so why can't you have the sleep equivalent to motivate and support you? After all, your sleep is much more important than some actor's bulging biceps!

 Top Tip: Don't be afraid to talk to someone you trust and ask their advice about your situation.

I'm not sure if I can do this

Your confidence is vital in changing the sleep habits of your children. If you look and act sheepish, your baby won't trust that you know what you're doing. And it's not difficult to see the reasons why parents' confidence sometimes wobbles. Half of what your mum did when you were a baby is now scientifically proven to be unhealthy, and what your dad or grandad probably did on the day his child was born (sit outside the

170

labour ward with the paper and a fag) is now totally taboo! However, sleep habits need to be tackled with certainty, so have confidence in yourself. *You can do it!* It's going to be so satisfying when you look back over your successes. You'll kick yourself for not having done it sooner! 'Why didn't we do it months ago?' is a familiar cry from parents who are now members of glowing, happily rested families.

Yes, I'm desperate and willing

Parents who are cheesed off with constantly disrupted nights fall into two camps:

- Desperate and willing to try anything. It's the desperate urgency of this condition which gives you the energy and the determination to be consistent in the tough times (i.e. at 3 a.m. when you're on the 257th visit to her cot that night).
- Don't like the way things are but haven't got the energy or interest to change. If this one applies to you, I'm afraid you're likely to fail before you've hardly started. So wait for a while until you're really, really desperate and then start again.

Dedication and consistency . . . that's what you need

Barry works as a long-distance lorry driver, travelling abroad for weeks at a time. Jean, his wife, looks after their two children, who are three and five years old. They both cry for attention at night, and Jean finds this really difficult to handle. When Barry is away she often lets them come into her bed at night. They don't cry and they both sleep well.

When Barry comes home, he and Jean argue, as Barry doesn't like the children in his bed. He often ends up sleeping on the sofa because there's not enough room in the bed with all of them. He misses the chance of being close to Jean and is resentful of the fact that the children's needs come before his. Jean just needs to get some undisrupted sleep and doesn't care how she gets it.

Sorting out sleep difficulties can be easier if you are a single parent, because you can be consistent in the way you set up sleep routines. In families where parents disagree, it is vital to discuss the differences, agree on a common, set way of dealing with bedtimes and night-waking, and present a united, consistent front to your child.

> **Top Tip:** *Changing sleep habits really is possible – especially if you are committed and appear confident.*

Sleep first, then the housework . . .

Sleep deprivation will take its toll on you. So before you set out to change your child's sleep habits, make life as easy as you can for yourself – stock up your cupboards with easy meals and decide to keep the washing, ironing, cooking and cleaning to a minimum. Ask everyone you know to help practically, and take it easy on yourself.

The bed's too big without you

There are all sorts of reasons why now might not be the right time to try to change your child's sleep patterns. Some of them may be to do with you. For instance, if you are facing difficult times, such as a bereavement, having your child in bed with you can be a real comfort.

Don't feel rushed into changing sleep habits unless you really want to. There are good and bad times for tackling sleep disruptions, so don't be tempted to go ahead when the time's not right.

> **Top Tip:** *Sometimes sleep problems need to be put on the back burner for a while, but once the time is right, don't delay – go for it! You'll be glad you did!*

Deeper issues

For some parents, bed-sharing with their child is a way to distance themselves from other things that are going on in their lives or to avoid talking about something important. Maybe you are having difficulty with your partner. Does one of you want your child in your bed so that the possibility of being honest, getting close to each other, being affectionate or making love becomes difficult or impossible? If you think this is the case, try to talk with your partner about it and listen to how they feel. This might mean facing up to other areas in your family life that you find difficult to deal with, but admitting to these feelings together is a start to a better, more honest relationship.

Once you talk more honestly together, your chances of successfully tackling your child's sleep problems are much higher. And as soon as your nights are less disturbed, you'll have more energy to face up to other problems you might be facing. You'll probably also start enjoying your child more, which, in turn, is likely to result in improvements in her daytime behaviour – and this, of course, will have added positive effects on you.

I'm not going to ask you to hop on to a black couch and go into deep psychotherapy here, but if you recognise that the sleep problem you're facing goes deeper than just your child, please find someone you trust to talk to. Try Parentline Plus (their phone number is at the back of this book), your health visitor or GP. Talking to someone about how you feel is half the battle. It may be terribly un-British, but it's likely to make you feel tons better.

 Top Tip: *If you suspect that there may be deeper issues behind the sleep problems you're facing, don't hesitate to talk to someone about it.*

Knowing when to get help

Despite reading all the books, buying all the T-shirts and trying all the theories, some sleep problems can be like stubborn stains, that nothing – not even Daz Ultra – is able to shift. This is also the time to get some outside help. Your first step should be your health visitor, though if your child has medical problems associated with sleep see your GP as well. Some GPs and health visitors are more interested in sleep behaviour than others; if yours isn't particularly helpful or isn't able to answer your questions, don't be frightened to ask if there is anyone else they know of locally who has a particular interest in sleep and who you could talk to. Increasingly, health visitors are setting up sleep clinics around the country. If there isn't one in your area you could even suggest they start one!

They're ready at the starting line . . . and they're off!

So you've got your plan sorted. Your child's going to stay in his bed all night. You've agreed with your partner when to start. Your mates are coming round with meals for the first three evenings and your child's looking worried!

'What, no more sleeping in bed all night with Daddy hanging half off the mattress?'

'No, but big cuddles and stories in bed in the morning.'

But be warned – you might turn into a 'sleep bore' and start coming out with phrases like 'It's changed my life. It's really incredible. You really should try it now!'

The best way to enjoy your children while they're young is to make sure that you have the sleep you need to be a good parent and that they get the sleep they need to be a good child. So decide what you'd like to change about your family's sleeping habits now. Plan how to go about achieving your goals and take the plunge. Be consistent, and you'll see the difference! Don't put it off. You need your sleep to be the best parent you can be, and 'because', as the woman in the shampoo commercial says, 'you're worth it!'

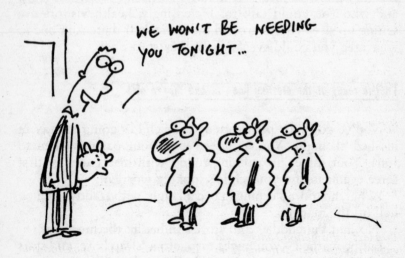

Further Information

Organisations

Parentalk
PO Box 23142
London SE1 OZT

Tel: 0700 2000 500
Fax: 020 7450 9060
e-mail: info@parentalk.co.uk
Web site: www.parentalk.co.uk

*Provides a range or resources and
services designed to inspire parents
to enjoy parenthood.*

Association for Postnatal Illness
145 Dawes Road
Fulham
London SW6 7EB

Tel: 020 7386 0868
Fax: 020 7386 8885
e-mail: info@apni.org
Web site: www.apni.org

*Provides information, advice and
support for women suffering from
postnatal illness.*

Care for the Family
PO Box 488
Cardiff CF15 7YY

Tel: 029 2081 0800
Fax: 029 2081 4089
e-mail: care.for.the.family@cff.org.
uk
Web site: www.care-for-the-family.
org.uk

*Providing support for families
through seminars, resources and
special projects.*

Community Health Council
National office
Association of Commumity Health
Councils for England and Wales
Earlsmead House
30 Drayton Park
London N5 1PB

Tel: 020 7609 8405
Fax: 020 7700 1152
e-mail: mailbox@achew.org.uk

*Look in the phone book for your
local branch – they can tell you
which GPs are working in your
area, and can put you in touch with
your local health visitor.*

CRY-SIS
BM CRY-SIS
London WC1N 3XX

Tel: 020 7404 5011 (8 a.m.–11 p.m.)
Web site:www.our-space.co.uk/serene.htm

Helpline for parents who are having problems with their children.

Down's Syndrome Association
In England:
155 Mitcham Road
London SW17 9PG
Tel: 020 8682 4001 (Tues–Thurs 10 a.m.–4 p.m.)

In Northern Ireland:
Graham House
Knockenbracken Healthcare Park
Saintfield Road
Belfast BT8 8BH
Tel: 028 9070 4606

In Wales:
206 Whitchurch Road
Cardiff CF14 3NB
Tel: 029 2052 2511
Web site: www.dsa-uk.com

Fathers Direct
Tamarisk House
37 The Tele Village
Crickhowell
Powys NP8 1BP

Tel: 01873 810 515
Web site: www.fathersdirect.com

Information resource for fathers.

The Foundation for the Study of Infant Deaths
14 Halkin Street
London SW1X 7DP

24-hour helpline: 020 7233 2090
Web site: www.sids.org.uk

Provides cot death research and support, including the Care of the Next Infant (CONI) scheme for parents who have lost a baby by SIDS.

Gingerbread
16–17 Clerkenwell Close
London EC1R OAA

Tel: 020 7336 8183
Fax: 020 7336 8185
e-mail: office@gingerbread.org.uk
Web site: www.gingerbread.org.uk

Provides day-to-day support and practical help for lone parents.

National Asthma Campaign
Providence House
Providence Place
London N1 0NT

Tel: 020 7226 2260
Helpline: 0845 701 0203 (run by nurses 9 a.m.–7 p.m.)
Web site: www.asthma.org.uk

The National Asthma Campaign is the independent UK charity working to conquer asthma, in partnership with people with asthma and all who share their concern, through a combination of research, education and support.

The National Autistic Society
393 City Road
London EC1V 1NG

Tel: 0870 600 8585
Autism helpline: 020 7903 3555
(Mon–Fri 10 a.m.–4 p.m.)
Parent to Parent helpline:
0800 9520 520 (your call is logged
onto an answer-phone and the
relevant regional volunteer will call
you back)
e-mail: autismhelpline@nas.org.uk
Web site: www.oneworld.org/
autism-uk

National Council for One Parent Families
255 Kentish Town Road
London NW5 2LX

Lone Parent Line: 0800 018 5026
Maintenance & Money Line: 020
7428 5424
(Mon & Fri 10.30 a.m.–1.30 p.m.;
Wed 3–6 p.m.)
Web site: www.oneparentfamilies.
org.uk

Information service for lone parents.

The National Eczema Society
Hill House
Highgate Hill
London N19 5NA

Information line: 0870 241 3604
(weekdays 1–4 p.m.)
General enquiries tel: 020 7281 3553
Web site: www.eczema.org

*The National Eczema Society is the
only charity in the UK dedicated to*

*providing support and information
for people with eczema and their
carers.*

National Family and Parenting Institute
430 Highgate Studios
53–79 Highgate Road
London NW5 1TL

Tel: 020 7424 3460
Fax: 020 7485 3590
e-mail: info@nfpi.org
Web site: www.nfpi.org

*An independent charity set up to
provide a strong national focus on
parenting and families in the
twenty-first century.*

NSPCC
NSPCC National Centre
42 Curtain Road
London EC2A 3NH

Tel: 020 7825 2500
Helpline: 0800 800 500
Fax: 020 7825 2525
Web site: www.nspcc.org.uk

*Aims to prevent child abuse and
neglect in all its forms and give
practical help to families with
children at risk. The NSPCC also
produces leaflets with information
and advice on positive parenting –
for these, call 020 7825 2500.*

Parentline Plus
520 Highgate Studios
53–79 Highgate Road
Kentish Town
London NW5 1TL

Helpline: 0808 800 2222
Textphone: 0800 783 6783
Fax: 020 7284 5501
e-mail: centraloffice@parentline
plus.org.uk
Web site: www.parentlineplus.org.
uk

*Provides a freephone helpline called
Parentline and courses for parents
via the Parent Network Service.
Parentline Plus also includes the
National Stepfamily Association. For
all information, call the Parentline
freephone number: 0808 800 2222.*

Parents Anonymous
6–9 Manor Gardens
London N7 6LA

Tel: 020 7263 8918 (Mon–Fri)

*24-hour answering service for
parents who feel they can't cope or
feel they might abuse their children.*

Positive Parenting
2A South Street
Gosport PO12 1ES

Tel: 023 9252 8787
Fax: 023 9250 1111
e-mail: info@parenting.org.uk
Web site: www.parenting.org.uk

*Aims to prepare people for the role
of parenting by helping parents,
those about to become parents and
also those who lead parenting
groups.*

Smoking Quitline
Helpline: 0800 002200

Twins and Multiple Birth Association
Harnott House
309 Chester Road
Ellesmere Port
Cheshire CH66 1QQ

Tel: 0870 1214000
Helpline 01732 868000 (Mon–Fri 7–
11 p.m.; weekends 10 a.m.–11 p.m.)
e-mail: enquiries@tambahq.org.uk
web site: www.tamba.org.uk

*Information and support to families
with twins, triplets and more.*

Publications

Toddler Taming, Dr Christopher Green, Vermillion
My Child Won't Sleep, Jo Douglas and Naomi Richman, Penguin Books
The Little Terror Good Sleeping Guide, Charlotte Preston and Trevor Dunton, Metro Books
Solve Your Child's Sleep Problems, Dr Richard Ferber, Dorling Kindersley
Your Baby and Child, Penelope Leach, Penguin Books
Raising Happy Children, Jan Parker and Jan Stimpson, Hodder and Stoughton

Parenting Courses

- **Parentalk Parenting Course**
  A new parenting course designed to give parents the opportunity to share their experiences, learn from each other and discover some principles of parenting. To find out more, contact:

  Parentalk
  PO Box 23142
  London SE1 0ZT

  Tel: 0700 2000 500
  e-mail: info@parentalk.co.uk
  Web site: www.parentalk.co.uk

- **Positive Parenting**
  Publishes a range of low-cost, easy-to-read, common sense resource materials which provide help, information and advice. Responsible for running a range of parenting courses across the UK. For more information phone 023 9252 8787.

- **Parent Network**
  For more information, call Parentline Plus on 0808 800 2222.

The **Paren**Talk Parenting Course

Helping you to be a Better Parent

Being a parent is not easy. **Parentalk** is a new, video-led, parenting course designed to give groups of parents the opportunity to share their experiences, learn from each other and discover some principles of parenting. It is suitable for anyone who is a parent or is planning to become a parent.

The Parentalk Parenting Course features:

Steve Chalke – TV Presenter; author on parenting and family issues; father of four and **Parentalk** Chairman.
Rob Parsons – author of *The Sixty Minute Father* and *The Sixty Minute Mother*; and Executive Director of Care for the Family.
Dr Caroline Dickinson – inner city-based GP and specialist in obstetrics, gynaecology and paediatrics.
Kate Robbins – well-known actress and comedienne.

Each **Parentalk** session is packed with group activities and discussion starters.

Made up of eight sessions, the **Parentalk** Parenting Course is easy to use and includes everything you need to host a group of up to ten parents.

Each Parentalk Course Pack contains:
- A **Parentalk** video
- Extensive, easy-to-use, group leader's guide
- Ten copies of the full-colour course material for members
- Photocopiable sheets/OHP masters

Price £49.95

Additional participant materials are available so that the course can be run again and again.

To order your copy, or to find out more, please contact:

ParenTalk
PO Box 23142, London SE1 0ZT
Tel: 0700 2000 500
Fax: 020 7450 9060
e-mail: info@parentalk.co.uk